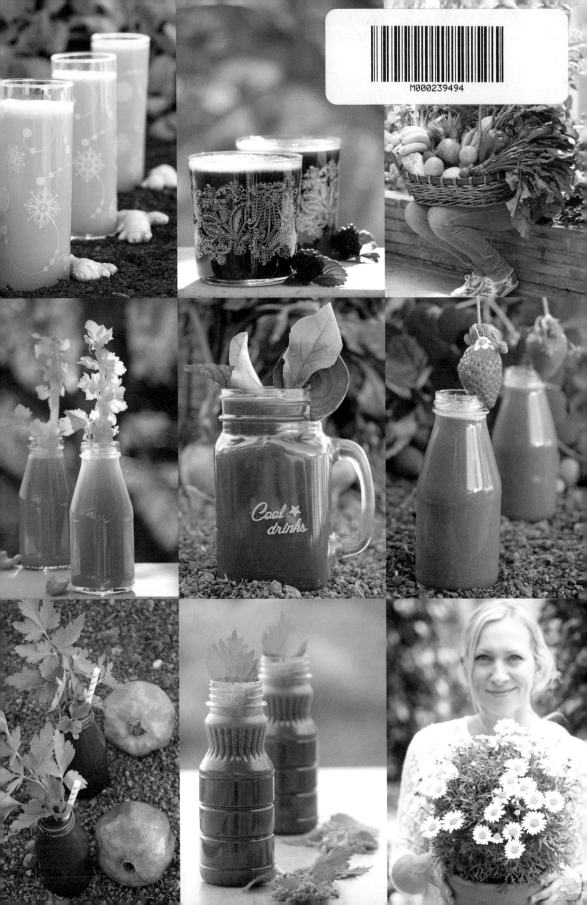

DETOX
SMOOTHIES

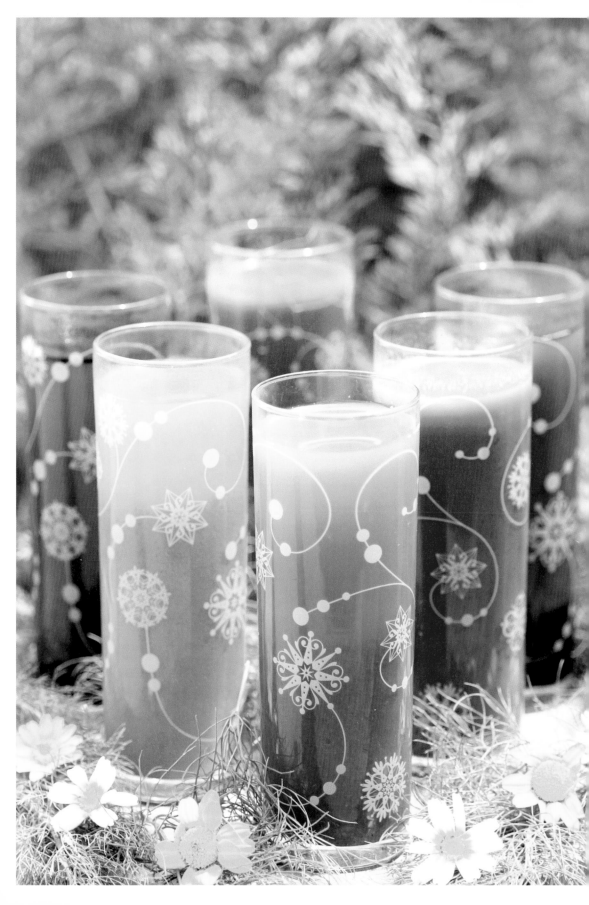

ELIQ MARANIK

DETOX SMOOTHIES

Lose Weight with Smoothies and Juices

h.f.ullmann

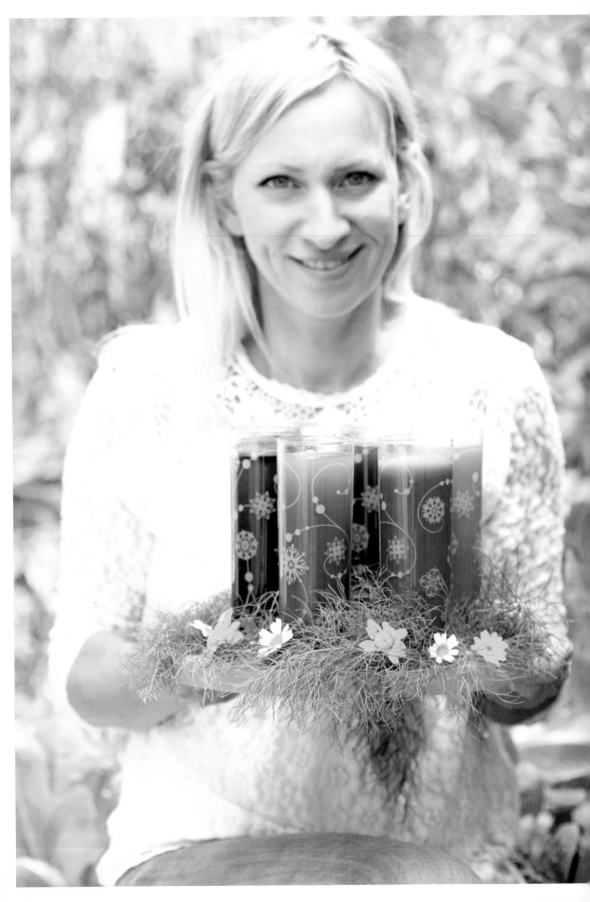

TABLE OF CONTENTS

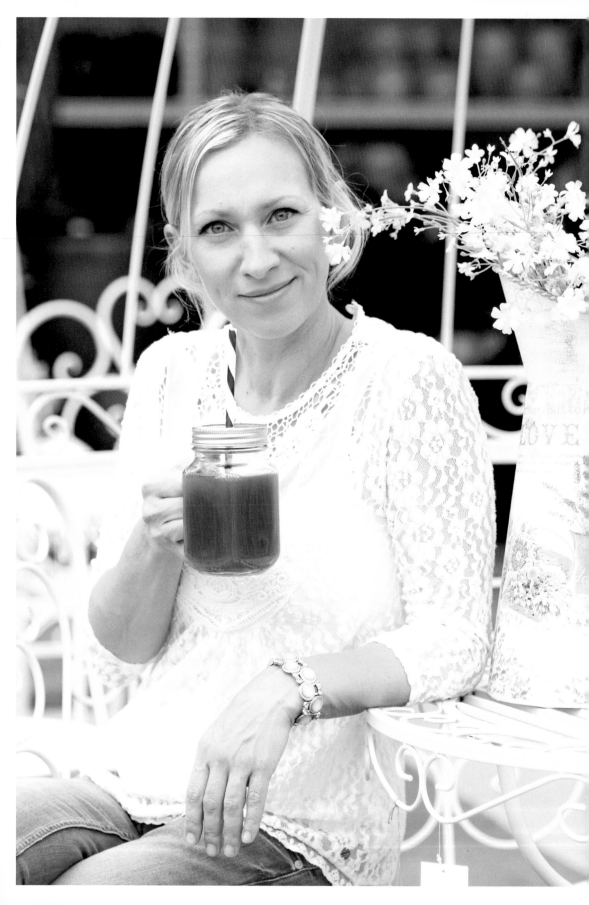

FOREWORD

Do you lack energy? Are you tired and feeling out of sorts? Is your digestion not functioning as it should? If so, it may be time to do a detox—and weight loss will come as an added bonus.

In this book I explore the basics of a detox: how you need to prepare, what you should think about during and after a detox, common side effects, what you can eat, and what foods you should steer clear of—all to help your body cleanse itself.

You don't necessarily need to do a hardcore detox—adding detoxifying nutrients to your diet will take you a long way—and there's nothing easier and healthier than making your own vegetable and fruit juices, smoothies, and nut shakes.

My very best juice and smoothie recipes are guaranteed to supply your body with clean energy and nutrients that will make you feel more energetic, happier, and healthier. Those who are curious can also read about how they can give their drinks an added boost with superfoods, how to make nut milks, and how to sprout at home.

The recipes are divided into three sections: Green and red juices and smoothies, Wellness shots, and Nut shakes and filling smoothies.

I hope I will inspire you to live a healthier and longer life.

Eliq Maranik

PLEASE NOTE: Pregnant and breastfeeding women, as well as those who are ill or who are feeling generally unwell, should never go on a detox.

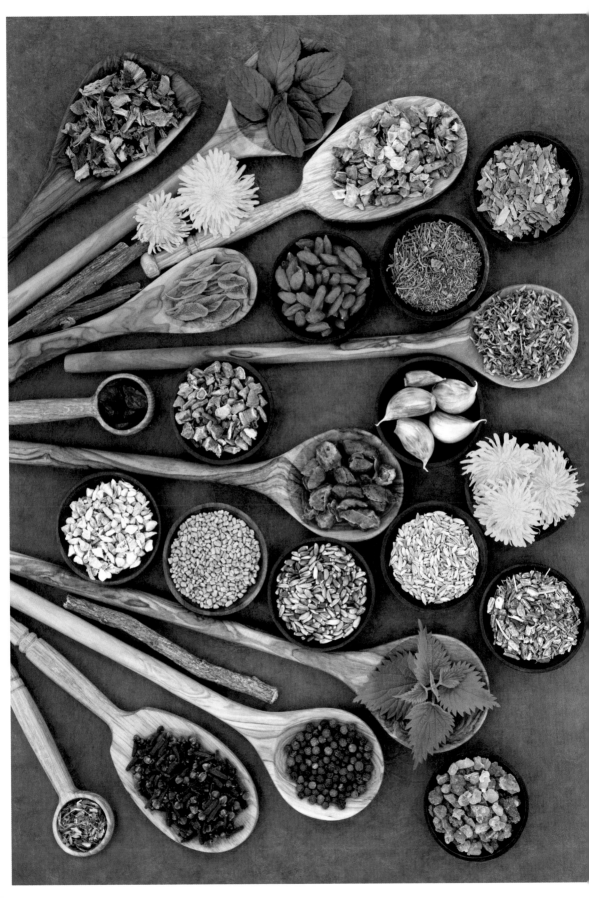

WHAT IS A DETOX?

A detox is a dietary program that promotes the elimination of toxins and waste products from the system, making you feel well and more alert, and giving you smoother skin and shinier hair, a properly functioning digestive system, and a stronger immune system. The word "detox" itself derives from the word "detoxification."

Through the ages, people have fasted and regularly cleansed their bodies in order to give them a chance to recover and detoxify. Detoxing means using various agents to actively encourage the function of those organs in the body that cleanse and detoxify it, for example using herbs that have a strengthening, cleansing, and regenerating effect. Vitamins, minerals, and antioxidants are another important part of a detox program.

To be on a detox diet means to give your body a "rest" for a period of time by excluding as many toxins as possible and eating a diet that is cleansing and full of antioxidants. This helps the body eliminate both toxins and waste products.

A detox regimen does not need to be dramatic or extreme, nor does it need to be unpleasant or painful. It is quick and easy to add green juices to your diet and eliminate "the worst offenders." The program should not be so strict as to make you desperately crave a hamburger or a piece of chocolate. The idea is to give your body a bit of a break and to reload on effective energy that will help your system to recover.

Every single day the body goes through its own physiological detoxification process—meaning that you sweat, pee, and poop, among other things. But in this day and age, where the world is full of pollution, heavy metals, radiation from computers, cell phones, microwave ovens, cigarettes, strong home-cleaning products, industrial effluents, chemical pesticides, alcohol, and a whole lot more, the body is exposed to many different kinds of toxins. Every now and then it needs a little help and,—most importantly—you need to learn to keep your body relatively toxin-free and change your bad habits.

KICKSTART TO A HEALTHY LIFESTYLE
A detox diet often serves as a kickstart to a new, healthy lifestyle. One reason for this is that as a result of detoxing you become aware of the importance of a balanced and, above all, healthy diet and of excluding foods that are bad for your body. A detox may also contribute to long-term weight loss. In today's world, most people not only eat the wrong foods but eat too much, and this results in the body becoming overburdened and ceasing to function with optimal efficiency. A detox will help to boost your digestive system and, in the long term, encourage you to adopt a healthy lifestyle.

TOXINS AND WASTE PRODUCTS
A lot of the food we eat contains substances that leave toxins and waste products in our bodies. These substances include trans fats, sugar, additives, pesticides, food colorings, and preservatives. But food is not the only culprit since waste products are also derived from external agents, such as exhaust fumes, emissions, or cigarette smoke. The body has an amazing ability to cleanse itself and manage smaller amounts of waste products and toxins. But when the quantities of waste products become too great and our systems become overburdened, the body is no longer able to take care of cleansing on its own. The liver, kidneys, intestines, and lymphatic system are detoxification organs that should work as effectively as they can. For example, if your liver is put under too much pressure, toxins might end up in your bloodstream and result

in symptoms such as fatigue, inflammation, swelling, sweating, and headache. Moreover, certain toxins and waste products can be stored in the body for years as the body is unable to get rid of them.

A detox diet helps to scoop up and eliminate toxins from the body. While you can buy various detox or similar products from health food stores, the single most important thing is to change your diet. Exclude toxins from your diet and, instead, eat a powerfully cleansing diet that consists of large quantities of fresh vegetables and fruits. Detox only a few times a year and you will come a long way by adding clean, healing energy to your body in the form of juice and smoothies and by excluding the worst offending foods, e.g. fully or half-processed foods, red meat, coffee, black tea, alcohol, and sugar. Read more on pages 15–17.

HELP YOUR BODY TO CLEANSE ITSELF

Lacking energy? Tired and lethargic? Digestive system not working as it should? If so, you may be in need of a detox lasting several days or several weeks. Detoxing need not mean feeling hungry all the time—on the contrary, you should ideally have two to three meals a day as well as several snacks. Drink green juices and replace some meals with a filling smoothie. You will learn to recognize the signs: of hunger; of when you have eaten enough; and also of when you should avoid eating through boredom, anxiety, or stress. Drink plenty of water, take exercise, and make sure that your body gets lots of vitamins, minerals, and antioxidants.

Beneficial effects of a detox diet:

» Your body will be cleansed of toxins and heavy metals.

» You will have more energy, feel happier, think more clearly, and have a better memory.

» Your immune system will improve.

» Your skin will become soft and smooth and less dry. You will look younger too!

» You will have stronger and more beautiful hair and nails.

» Problems from bloating, gas, and abdominal pain will be minimized or disappear.

» Your metabolism and energy-burning capacity will improve.

» Your mood will be more stable.

» You will lose weight.

» Your cells will repair and regenerate.

» Your stomach and intestines will start working more efficiently because your body will be given time to rest and because you will be introducing beneficial bacteria through your improved diet.

» You will sleep more soundly and experience less stress.

» You will have fewer or less severe colds.

» In most cases, your pain, joint pain, and allergies will improve.

DO YOU NEED A DETOX?

The body stores undesirable substances and toxins in its fat cells. It is perfectly possible for someone to walk around with up to 11 extra pounds / 5 kg of unhealthy, slimy, toxic waste.

We live in a world that is full of potential toxins in the water we drink, the food we eat, and the air we breathe. The body's organs are affected by how we live, and our lifestyles may cause imbalances that lead to health problems. Difficulty sleeping, headaches, and other pain may improve or even completely disappear on a detox program. Another positive thing is that your body is itself capable of quickly ridding itself of toxins if you only help it along.

- » Do you have frequent headaches or migraines?
- » Do you often feel tired, feel rough, and have problems concentrating?
- » Do you get more than three colds, bouts of flu, or other viral infections during the course of an average year?
- » Do you often get fungal infections?
- » Has your sex drive decreased?
- » Do you have bad breath or an acid reflux?
- » Do you often have stomach ache, digestive problems, a bloated or gassy stomach?
- » Is your skin dry, red-blotched, puffy, and/or swollen?
- » Do you have fertility problems?
- » Do you often eat frozen and/or convenience foods?

- » Do you regularly use tobacco products?
- » Do you often drink coffee or black tea?
- » Do you often drink alcohol?
- » Do you often consume sugar in the form of candy, baked rolls, and white bread?
- » Do you take medication, painkillers, or other chemical preparations?
- » Do you live near areas where the air is polluted?
- » Are you not having a daily bowel movement?
- » Are you overweight?
- » Do you have sleeping problems?
- » Do you often feel unhappy, negative, or depressed?

HOW LONG AND HOW OFTEN SHOULD YOU DETOX?

Everyone should decide for themselves what the extent and frequency of their detox program will be. It is important that you listen to your body and do not press yourself too hard if you are unused to detoxing. If you have never detoxed before, you should start with a program lasting one to three days. If you have more experience in detoxing, set yourself a period of three to seven days. If you feel ready to go on a hard-core detox, you can extend this period up to a month. Find the most suitable solution for you and always adjust your detox according to how you are feeling.

Anyone can go on a one-day detox and reap benefits from it. A three-day detox is a great idea because, in that space of time, your body will have the time to eliminate all the "white toxins," such as sugar, gluten, and milk. If you want to do a "proper" detox, a week to ten days is perfectly adequate, but you should prepare your body for the detox and treat it kindly afterward.

You can do one to two intensive detox programs a year, one in the spring and one in the fall. During such a program, you focus on an intensive 7–28-day elimination of all the chemicals, heavy metals, and other waste products from your body and allow your body to cleanse itself by giving the digestion less work to do.

First of all, choose the type of detox you want to do: a full fast, a half fast, only eating raw foods, eating everything apart from "the forbidden foods," having colonic irrigation, going to saunas, dry-brushing your skin, or taking regular detox baths? Feel free to combine several of these methods. You also need to decide how long you want to detox for. Start your program on a Thursday or Friday, especially if you are not used to fasting or detoxing, as this will allow you to rest a little more during the weekend.

The best way for first-time detoxers to ease themselves into their chosen program is to eliminate certain foods (see page 17) and to top up on pure energy by drinking green juices and herbal teas and by going to the sauna or taking a detox bath (see pages 19, 20). Rethinking your food and eating a healthy diet is the best thing you can do for your body in the long term. However, treating yourself to an occasional unnecessary treat is absolutely fine.

PREPARING FOR A DETOX

To make the most of your detox, you should prepare yourself mentally and physically for it. Set aside a non-busy period when you will have time to rest, and start on a weekend. Take it easy and give your body more time to rest than you would usually do. Equally, make sure you do not work out as much as you normally do—go for long walks instead. Empty your pantry and refrigerator and top up on detox-friendly foods, such as fresh vegetables, fruits, nuts, and seeds. Go for locally produced and organic food in order to minimize your exposure to pesticides. A few days to a week before you start with your detox program, you would do well to reduce or entirely exclude alcohol, tobacco, coffee, black tea, and fully and semi-processed foods from your diet in order to allow your body to get used to the change. Drink at least four to six pints / 2–3 liters of water every day so that your body can flush itself out. Start your day with a large glass of lukewarm water containing the juice of a freshly squeezed lemon, as this helps to cleanse your intestines.

For detox beginners or people who need additional support, it may be helpful to visit a detox center or health resort with a friend. You should never go on a detox if you are pregnant or breastfeeding, or if you are sick or feeling generally unwell. In that case, you should consult your doctor before making any major changes to your diet.

A FEW TIPS BEFORE YOU START YOUR DETOX:

1. Prepare for your detox
The first few days of a detox can be hard and you may feel tired, have a cold or headache, or feel generally unwell as your body gets ready to eliminate the toxins. You may also experience withdrawal symptoms, which is due to both your brain and your body having to give up the toxins they have become used to on a daily basis. That is why it is a good idea to start your detox on a Friday so that you do not have to struggle through the most difficult symptoms while you are at work. Tell people around you that you are doing a detox—hopefully, they will be sympathetic and understand better what you are going through.

2. Make sure you are psyched up before you start
Choose a period in your life when you feel well-balanced and when things are fine. Starting a detox at a time when you are struggling with a heavy workload, worries, or difficulties may prove problematic and result in your feeling worse and even more stressed.

3. Detox with a friend
It is both easier and more fun to detox with one or more good friends. You give each other support and everyone goes through the same process. Compliment both yourself and your friends on your efforts—being positive will make everyone feel more positive!

4. Do not neglect your snacks
During a detox you should feel that it is easy and natural to focus on your diet and wellbeing. Make sure you do not neglect your snacks. Remember, you will be more likely to give up if you are feeling hungry.

5. Cut down on your workout time
Working out during a detox is fine, but make sure you do not push yourself as much as you normally would. Avoid high-intensity exercise and do yoga, pilates, or stretching exercises or go for long walks instead. Find out what works for you so you know what your body is most comfortable with. The most important thing is that you feel your body is getting more energy from your workout. There is no point in getting tired and having little energy after a workout. If you push your body too hard, it will be screaming for unhealthy foods.

6. Take it easy

Make sure that your schedule is not too busy when you are detoxing. It would be great if you could slow down a little, especially for the first few days. Start on a Friday so that you can concentrate on your detox for the first weekend and spend it in peace and quiet. Try to find inner peace and focus on your body and what you put into it. Make time for yourself, relax, go for a walk in the countryside, take a warm bath, go for a sauna or a spa, get a massage or two, and spend time with yourself. Avoid negative thoughts and people who make you feel bad.

7. Get more sleep

Go to bed early and get a good night's sleep—at least eight to nine hours. Besides, sleeping an hour longer may help you lose weight. When you are stressed, your body secretes hormones that slow down your metabolism. Never feel guilty about getting enough sleep or taking it easy.

8. Drink water

You should drink at least four to six pints / 2–3 liters of water each day. This can include herbal teas and lemon water. The water you drink should preferably be at body temperature, i.e. 97–98.6 °F / 37–38 °C.

COMMON SIDE EFFECTS

Most people experience weight loss during a detox, but you may find that your mood is also delicate and sensitive. You may have to deal with different emotions that come to the surface, or you may find yourself thinking about what you want to do with the rest of your life. Some people cry a lot during a detox, while others become angry or are brimming with joy.

Mild detox symptoms such as fatigue, headaches, mood swings, frequent urination, and feeling emotionally aloof are common during the first few days. These are signs that your body is responding to the detox, so the more stressed you are, the tougher it can be. Headaches are often caused by caffeine, so it is a good idea to give up coffee even before you start your detox. If you find that you are experiencing too many withdrawal symptoms, you could scale down your program for a little while and then step it up again a day or two later. If you are really out of sorts or experience pain somewhere in your body, you should stop your detox and consult your doctor. You can also get good advice and guidance from a nutritionist or an experienced health coach. The purpose of a detox is to supply you with energy, not to make you feel troubled or suffer from poor health.

WHAT TO DO AFTER YOUR DETOX

When you finish your detox, it is extremely important that you try to maintain healthy eating habits. If you immediately go back to your old habits, you will easily stress out your body and your health could be worse than it was. Listen to your body: it is talking to you!

Slowly increase your food intake, making sure that you take your time and that you give your body the time to get used to the new situation. Start slowly and pay close attention to how food is affecting you. If you eat something that results in symptoms such as fatigue, depression, heaviness in the body, headache, or stomach problems, it may be helpful to avoid these foods for a shorter or longer period of time.

Many people feel much better and revise their attitudes to food during and after a detox. It also makes it easier for them to work out which foods make them feel good and which do not. When your body is completely clean, you will find it easy to work out which foods give you stomachache and which foods make you feel more energetic.

After a detox you will feel more healthy and lighter—and you will have a lot of energy. In addition, your immunity will have improved and your body will be better equipped to fight colds and similar illnesses.

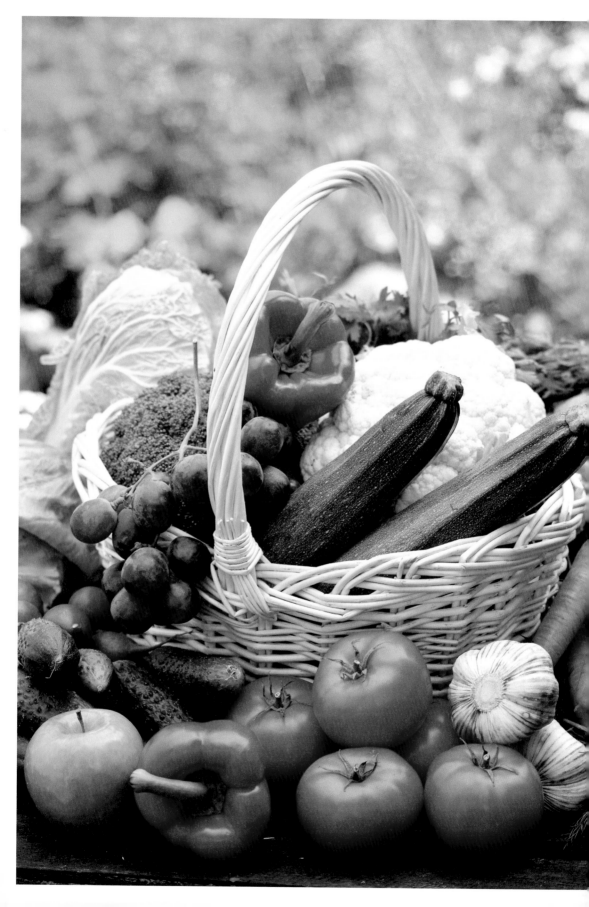

WHAT TO EAT WHEN YOU ARE DETOXING

The primary aim of this book is to offer you an abundance of tasty recipes for juices and smoothies that work well as part of a detox program, but it also teaches the basics of detoxing and its benefits for the body.

There are many different levels of detoxification, some being almost identical to fasting and allowing only drinks for energy, some allowing most things. Obviously, you do not necessarily need to choose the strictest detox program; you will go far by just excluding some foods from your diet (see the list on the next page) and replacing your breakfast, snack, and/or dinner with chlorophyll-rich vitamin bombs. The important thing is that you and your body feel good and that you feel energized from all the pure energy found in fruit and vegetables. I believe you should have at least one hot meal a day, or preferably more, so that you do not feel hungry and so that you do not get cravings, because it is easy to give up in such situations. You should decide what works for you.

Make sure you have some good herbal teas to hand as a replacement for those cups of coffee and tea you are used to having every day. Another good idea, if and when you get a craving, is to eat some unsalted, unroasted nuts, homemade snack bars, or vegetable sticks. During the day, you can have as much filtered water or herbal tea as you like. Good teas include nettle, dandelion, chamomile, mint, green tea, Ayurvedic herbal blends, ginger tea, and other natural, caffeine-free teas.

Remember to avoid, as much as possible, anything that contains gluten, sugar, lactose, e-numbers, and preservatives. Eat vegetarian food and bear in mind that you can get protein from legumes, mushrooms, and tofu products. Try to buy locally produced and organic produce.

The lists below contain examples of what you can eat during your detox and what you should avoid for your body to recover optimally. Hopefully, your detox program will also prove to be the beginning of a lifestyle that is a little healthier.

FRUIT AND VEGETABLES
» Leafy vegetables (e.g. spinach, chard, nettle, dandelion, curly endive, lamb's lettuce, escarole, radicchio, romaine lettuce, iceberg lettuce).
» Sprouts and shoots (e.g. alfalfa, fenugreek, mung beans, broccoli, radish, wheat, buckwheat, millet, quinoa, sunflower seeds, flaxseed, chia seeds, peas. For more information about sprouts, please see pages 39–40.)
» All varieties of cabbage (e.g. kale, white cabbage, red cabbage, broccoli, cauliflower, kohlrabi, Brussels sprouts, Savoy cabbage, pointed cabbage).
» Root vegetables (e.g. carrot, rutabaga, beet, radish, parsnip, celeriac, Jerusalem artichoke, horseradish, sweet potato).
» Stem vegetables (e.g. celery, fennel, artichoke, asparagus, avocado, corn).
» Fruit-bearing vegetables (e.g. cucumber, tomato, eggplant, bell pepper, pumpkin, squash, zucchini).
» Legumes (e.g. peas, beans, haricot beans, soy beans).
» Fruit (e.g. banana, pineapple, apple, pear, mango, papaya, kiwi, plum, apricot, nectarine, pomegranate, melon).
» Berries (fresh or frozen).
» Citrus fruit (e.g. grapefruit, lemon, lime, pomelo, orange, mandarin).

- » Onion, leek, garlic.
- » Fresh herbs and spices (e.g. ginger, turmeric, red chile, cilantro, mint, dill, chives, sage, parsley, rosemary, thyme).

FOR THE PANTRY

- » Lentils.
- » Garbanzo beans.
- » Beans.
- » Quinoa.
- » Millet.
- » Buckwheat.
- » Oats.
- » Amaranth.
- » Brown rice.
- » Brown rice noodles.
- » Polenta.
- » All types of nuts and seeds, natural and unroasted.
- » Dried fruit, organic and additive-free (but beware of the sugar content!).
- » Hemp seeds and hemp protein.
- » Organic miso soup, powder.
- » Algae, organic.
- » Organic broth, additive-free.
- » Dried herbs (e.g. turmeric, coriander, cumin, oregano, rosemary, thyme, paprika, black pepper, cloves, cardamom, cinnamon, nutmeg, saffron).
- » Cold-pressed, organic oils (e.g. coconut oil, olive oil, rapeseed oil).
- » Organic honey.
- » Peanut butter, organic.
- » Gluten-free flour (e.g. almond flour, coconut flour, psyllium husks, garbanzo meal, rice flour, buckwheat flour, oat flour, quinoa flour).
- » Natural sweeteners (e.g. organic, dried apricots, figs, dates, frozen banana, frozen mango, organic honey).
- » Superberries and superfoods (sea buckthorn powder, blueberry powder, raw cocoa).
- » Coconut milk, additive-free.

FOR THE REFRIGERATOR

- » Soy products (e.g. milk, yogurt, cream, tofu).
- » Oat products (e.g. milk, yogurt, cream).

ANIMAL PRODUCTS

If you want to do an extreme detox, you should exclude all foods derived from animal products. However, if you do decide to eat animal products, make sure they are organic because any animal that has not been reared organically is sure to have been fed hormones, antibiotics, and non-organic foods, which in your body convert to precisely the toxins and waste products that you want to get rid of.

» Organic eggs.

» Organic white meats (chicken and turkey).

» Fish (excluding tuna, swordfish, and farmed salmon).

» Buffalo mozzarella, goat cheese, feta cheese, ricotta, cottage cheese (made from milk other than cow's milk).

AN EXAMPLE OF A DETOX DAY:

20–30 minutes before breakfast: 1–2 pints / ½–1 liter of 98 °F / 37 °C degree filtered water, with freshly squeezed lemon or lime juice.

Breakfast: A green juice or smoothie.

Snack: A generous handful of nuts or almonds, soaked overnight.

Lunch: A hot vegetarian meal, the largest meal of the day.

Snack: An avocado and a handful of nuts, soaked overnight.

Dinner: A nut shake or a wholesome smoothie, or alternatively a vegetarian meal.

Late evening: Green juice.

During the day, you can drink as much filtered water and herbal tea as you like. If you are going to be working out, eat several small meals rather than one large one.

THINGS TO AVOID:

» Alcohol.

» Coffee, black tea, cola, and other caffeine-containing products.

» Nicotine.

» Sugar and sweets.

» White flour and white flour products.

» Salt.

» Sweeteners.

» Trans fats.

» E-numbers.

» Fully or semi-processed foods.

» "Lite" products.

» Red meat (which contains a lot of hormones injected into the animal to make it grow faster).

» Tuna, swordfish, freshwater fish.

» Chicken (if you are doing a strict detox, since it contains a lot of hormones injected into the animal to make it grow faster).

» Dairy products made from cow's milk. Instead, use products based on oats, soy, and nuts such as oat milk, nut milk, soy milk, and soy yogurt.

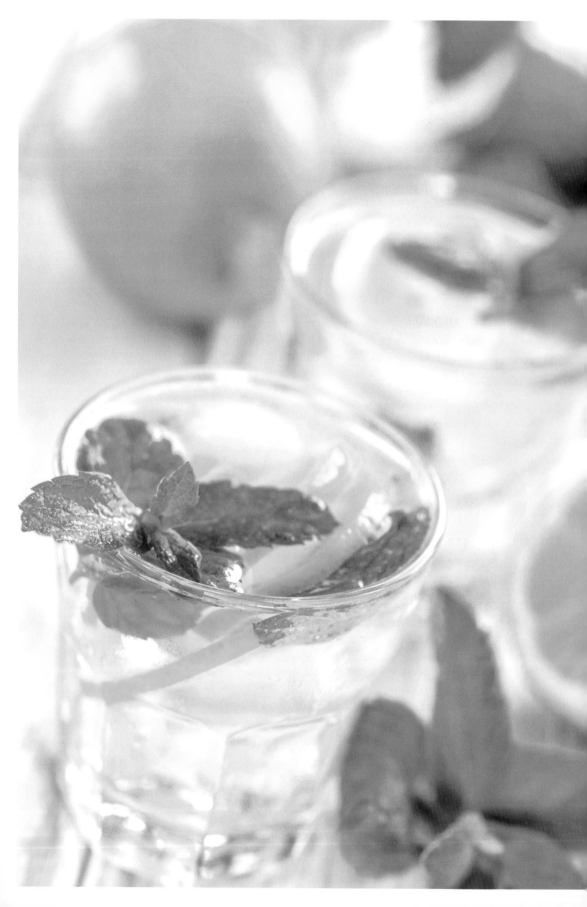

OTHER DETOX TIPS

START YOUR DAY WITH LEMON WATER

A perfect start to the day—before you step into the shower and get ready—is to alkalize your body by having a large glass of filtered water with freshly-squeezed lemon juice, 20–30 minutes before you eat or drink anything else. This will help to cleanse your bowels. In order to keep your body in an alkalized state, it may also be helpful to drink a glass of lemon water 20–30 minutes before each meal. The water should be roughly at body temperature.

ACTIVATED CHARCOAL

Activated charcoal is the world's oldest detoxifying agent. It has been used for centuries in Chinese, Ayurvedic, and Western medicine. Activated charcoal absorbs toxins and heavy metals in the body and suppresses bloating and flatulence. It is a highly absorbent material with millions of small pores that can trap and bind up to 100 times its own weight, which makes it an ideal agent for eliminating potentially toxic substances from your gastrointestinal tract.

In high doses, activated charcoal may cause constipation and make your stools dark. The charcoal absorbs all foreign substances, so never take activated charcoal with medication. Activated charcoal is available in pharmacies and health food stores.

SAUNA BATHING

Our bodies need some help to promote circulation, and sweating causes unwanted toxins and waste products to be released from the body.

Any form of sauna bathing is a powerful detoxification method because a good sweat activates the body's self-cleansing mechanisms. You can train your body to sweat more. Similarly, you can gradually get used to the heat if you are finding it a problem. Just bear in mind that this highly efficient form of detox is available and free of charge in every single fitness center!

Start by taking a shower and washing off all your makeup. Stay in the sauna as long as comfortable, taking a cooling shower from time to time. Drinking plenty of water can increase your body's natural ability to sweat, but do avoid bringing plastic bottles into the sauna because the heat can release chemicals into it.

You may feel a little sluggish and tired after a sauna because your body is hard at work cleansing itself. But if you take water and nutrients afterward, as well as some rest, you will feel amazing. Sauna bathing is the world's simplest detox method—it is absolutely fantastic if you want a healthy-looking and beautiful skin.

The beneficial effects of sauna bathing:

» Speeds up fat burning and eliminates toxins and waste products.

» Increases circulation to all body cells.

» Balances hormones and blood sugar.

» Improves mobility and reduces pain.

» Stimulates the immune system and inhibits viruses.

» Strengthens the nervous system and brain capacity.

» Lowers blood pressure and strengthens the heart.

» Increases the amount of pleasure-inducing endorphins.

» Ensures healthy-looking and beautiful skin.

DETOX BATHING

Detoxifying the body by taking a detox bath is an old home remedy. If you have a bathtub, take a detox bath in the comfort of your home. A detox bath is intended to help the body to eliminate toxins and absorb minerals and nutrients found in the water. You can buy natural products for a detox bath in health food stores, including soap and various types of bath salts. They should be free of colorants, perfumes, and preservatives.

I use *Sannas Såpa* for long detox baths. It is a natural product, without any synthetic surfactants, water softeners, preservatives, or perfumes, and is made from distilled tall oil that has been saponified with calcium hydroxide. This soap, which offers several health benefits to the skin, can also be used as a soap for the whole body. It is alkaline and fights harmful bacteria, fungi, and molds; it stimulates circulation and has a healing effect on itches, eczema, and acne; it is environmentally friendly and a little goes a long way; finally, it is gentle on the skin, deep-cleansing and moisturizing.

To prepare a long detox bath: Pour 1–1⅓ cups of soap into the bathtub, fill up with hot water and stay in the bath for one to three hours. Every now and then, drain off the water and refill the bathtub with more hot water. The bath has a detoxifying and rejuvenating effect. You will sleep like a baby afterward! Drink plenty of water at room temperature during and after the bath. Do a 3-week detox by taking three to four baths a week. If you feel sick or dizzy, you should immediately stop bathing and take a new bath some other time.

Remember to make it a pleasant experience—light some candles, put some relaxing music on or listen to a nice audiobook, meditate or ask a friend to join you for a chat while you are having the bath.

PSYLLIUM HUSKS

When you are constipated, faeces sit around in your gut and the toxins that are formed are absorbed by the intestinal mucosa, leading to self-poisoning. During a detox, you will need a lot of fiber in your diet so that toxins and waste products can be removed and your bowel movements work as they should. Psyllium husks absorb toxins and put your intestines to work in a gentle way. That makes them a simple solution for detoxers. When the husks reach the gut, the fiber forms a gelatinous mass—a type of bulking agent—that increases intestinal activity, which in turn counteracts constipation. It is good to take psyllium husks in the morning and evening in order to bind and eliminate the toxins from the gut. They also reduce hunger.

Remember to drink plenty of water when you eat psyllium husks as they are extremely rich in fiber. A common side effect is that they may cause stomach upset in the first few days. So, start with a small teaspoon to allow your body to get used to them. Soon, your stomach will stabilize and flatulence will diminish. Psyllium husks are available in well-stocked grocery stores and health food stores. If you can't get hold of psyllium husks, you can replace them with flaxseed or chia seeds.

DRY-BRUSHING YOUR SKIN

The lymphatic system consists of the lymph nodes and an extensive network of lymphatic vessels running throughout the whole body. Lymph removes toxins, waste products, and inflammations from the tissues. By dry-brushing your skin, you scrub off residues of old skin and stimulate your whole lymphatic system, which in turn facilitates the expulsion of waste products.

The skin itself is a large detoxification organ. Dry-brushing helps to keep your skin pores open and clean, and complements the detoxification work done by both the liver and the kidneys. The result is an improved immune system and healthier more supple skin.

You will need a brush made of natural fibers, neither too soft nor too bristly. Avoid synthetic brushes. Make dry-brushing your daily routine. It takes two to three minutes, depending on how much you want to stroke each area, and the result is fantastic.

Method: Use a dry brush. Your skin, too, should be dry so, ideally, make sure you brush before you take a shower in the morning. Brushing increases the blood flow and will help you wake up. Start with your feet. Always brush in the direction of the heart. Start with your feet and legs, brushing 5–10 times from the bottom up, the front and rear of your legs, as well as the inside and the outside. Brush upwards and across your legs with long, light and fast movements. Continue brushing from your fingertips, hands, arms, and up toward your shoulders, as well as inward toward your heart in the same fashion, 5–10 times, to encourage your blood to return to the heart and strengthen your lymphatic system. Brush your midriff area 5–10 times, using clockwise circular movements, and bear in mind that every time you brush, the stroke should be directed toward your heart. Avoid brushing your face, nipples, and any areas of irritated skin. Feel free to experiment. If you brush too forcefully, your skin will become red and irritated. Rinse your brush with water every couple of weeks and let it dry before using it again.

The benefits of dry-brushing your skin:

» Skin will become supple and will tighten up.

» Digestion will improve.

» Cellulite will decrease or disappear.

» Cell renewal will increase.

» Lymphatic system will work more efficiently.

» Dead skin cells will be removed.

» Immune system will be strengthened.

PROBIOTICS

Healthy intestinal flora is the foundation of good health. Probiotics are beneficial bacteria that are considered be very important for the intestinal flora and even for the immune system. The bacteria balance the microflora in the intestines, aiding digestion and detoxification. Probiotic bacteria compete with pathogenic intestinal bacteria for both nutrition and space. In the colon, probiotics assist in the creation of K and B vitamins, including B1, B2, B6, and B9, as well as various amino acids that promote mineral absorption. Probiotics are also extremely helpful for people with severe indigestion and for restoring intestinal flora balance during or after a course of antibiotics.

If you have had colonic irrigation (see below) in order to cleanse your body of impurities, harmful bacteria, toxins, any parasitic diseases, candida, and other conditions, you are at great risk of also having reduced the quantity of your beneficial bacteria. That is exactly why you need to top up on probiotics afterward. It is okay to take probiotics before your intestinal cleanse, but it is more common to do it immediately afterward.

Probiotics consist of strains of lactic bacteria or specific yeast cells, for example, various types of lactic bacteria, bifidobacteria, acidophilus bacteria, and *Streptococcus thermophilus*.

Probiotics can be taken in capsule, tablet, or drop form and are available in health food stores and pharmacies. Probiotics are also included in foods such as yogurt.

COLONIC IRRIGATION

Colonic irrigation is done by a professional practitioner who uses a special piece of equipment. You will see the contents of your gut pass into a glass tube, from where it is carried off direct into the sewers. The method is completely odorless and hygienic. Irrigation with water has a very positive effect on the intestines. Combining a detox with colonic irrigation produces a faster and more thorough-going effect. It is extremely important to top up on probiotics, beneficial intestinal bacteria, immediately after the session.

Colonic irrigation frees the intestines from the waste products that remain in the body after it has absorbed the nutrients from food. Unless you help your colon from time to time—especially if you have neglected your diet—some waste products will stay in your gut, making your stomach stressed and edgy and thereby causing problems. Colonic irrigation is a simple way of helping your body to cleanse and eliminate impurities left behind in your intestines. This means your stomach can get a bit of a rest and your body a chance to relax fully.

CHLOROPHYLL

The vital force that explodes into greenness in nature can be transferred to the human body through chlorophyll. When chlorophyll enters the body, the same thing happens as in the plant world—chlorophyll oxygenates, cleans, cleanses, and regenerates.

One of the major reasons why green plants are so beneficial to us is their chlorophyll, which is available in abundance in all green plants. Chlorophyll has a chemical structure similar to that of our own hemoglobin, which is why it helps to increase the transport of oxygen and nutrients to the body's cells. Chlorophyll has four main effects on our bodies: it is cleansing, it is regenerating, it fights inflammation, and it has a powerful detoxifying effect.

A simple way to consume a lot of chlorophyll is by drinking chlorophyll-rich juices made from green leaves and green vegetables or a teaspoon of spirulina, wheatgrass powder, barley grass powder, or any other chlorophyll-rich powder in a glass of water or juice. You will definitely notice the difference!

Make juices with ingredients you like. The only thing you should bear in mind is not to base your juices on fruit alone. Ideally, half or two-thirds of the juice you drink should consist of various vegetables, preferably dark green leaves. Beneficial vegetables include cucumber, celery, all kinds of cabbage, beets, fennel, spinach, broccoli, lemon, ginger, and all types of green leaves. Always buy organic, unsprayed vegetables. That way you won't be putting any additional toxins or waste products into your body.

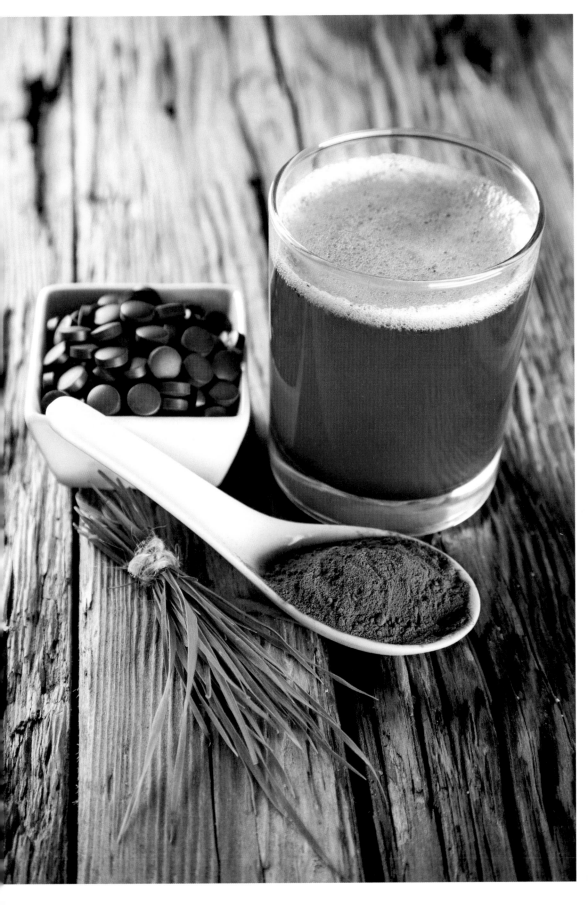

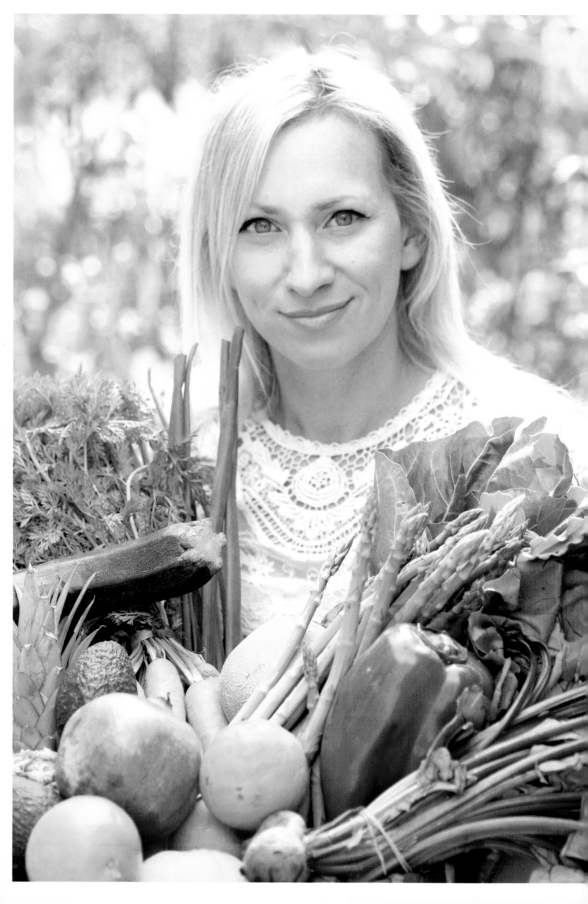

BUYING AND HANDLING FRUIT AND VEGETABLES

CHOOSE VEGETABLES, FRUIT, AND BERRIES WITH CARE

The art of successfully making tasty and healthy juices and smoothies starts when you are standing at the fruit and vegetable counter. Learning to find, choose, store, and use the produce of the season properly is all-important. The most useful method of finding absolutely the best produce is to use your eyes, nose, and fingers and, as far as possible, to buy that which is locally produced.

Local markets and direct farm sales offer the freshest produce in addition to usually being less expensive than your typical grocery store. There are also several savvy businesses that deliver fruit and vegetables straight to your door and that generally provide information about where their produce comes from, what varieties they are delivering and, sometimes, even grower's references.

BUY ORGANIC

Since you are trying to eliminate toxins from your body, most of the produce you are eating and drinking should be unsprayed, i.e. organic. Besides, organic fruit and vegetables contain more vitamins, minerals, enzymes, and other nutrients than those that are conventionally grown. Among other things, they have higher vitamin C and antioxidant levels.

WASH AND SCRUB

If the produce you are consuming is not organic, in the case of fruit, berries, or vegetables that have not been picked from your own garden you simply do not know how they have been treated, where they have been stored, and who has handled them—not to mention any spraying or waxing. Even fruit with an inedible skin, such as banana, orange, mandarin, melon, etc., should be washed properly because everything that is on your hands will pass into your body when you are handling the flesh of the fruit.

The simplest solution to this problem is to fill a mixing bowl with lukewarm water, add the juice of a lemon and a few tablespoonfuls of vinegar to it, and immerse your fruit, berries, vegetables, or lettuce in the water for 5 minutes. You then thoroughly wash and brush off all the hard-skinned fruits and vegetables under cold running water using a soft vegetable brush. Do not use this brush for any other purpose, and wash it thoroughly after each use. You can wash soft-skinned fruit by rubbing it with your hands or by using the soft part of a kitchen sponge (which you also only use to wash produce). Lettuce, berries, and other produce that is damaged easily should be rinsed with cold water after being soaked in lemony water. All the dirt will come right off, without the flavor being affected. You can also buy special organic-produce washes.

The safest way of handling non-organic fruit is to peel it.

TO PEEL OR NOT TO PEEL

The highest levels of vitamins, minerals, and enzymes are found just under the surface of or inside the skin of fruit and vegetables. If you consume organic produce, you should therefore, with a few exceptions, not peel the skin. Always peel or skin citrus fruit (bitter-tasting), all varieties of melons, bananas, mango, pineapple, and avocado. However, kiwi and papaya do not always need to be peeled—if you are going to juice them, leave the skin on, but if you are going to blend them, it is best to remove the skin first. Always remove the thinnest layer possible when peeling or skinning fruit and vegetables.

STONES

Remove the large stones of mango, avocado, nectarine, peach, plum, apricot, and other stone fruit. Soft pips and seeds, such as those of melon and watermelon, can be juiced, but I usually remove them when blending. Papaya seeds are very healthful but will impart a spicy, almost peppery, flavor to your juice or smoothie. Try it yourself and see what you think. A word of caution, though: refrain from eating large amounts of papaya if you are or want to become pregnant—in some countries, papaya is used as a natural means of birth control.

SERVE IMMEDIATELY

For optimal vitamin content, flavor, color, and consistency, you should serve smoothies and freshly squeezed juices as soon as possible after preparation. If you want to save your juice or smoothie for later, you can store it in a clean, closed glass bottle in the fridge, but ideally for no longer than 24 hours, because the vitamins will, slowly but surely, disappear and the contents will go off pretty quickly. Shake the bottle well before drinking your juice or smoothie.

I have a FoodSaver, a vacuum sealer machine, which comes with a lot of smart jars and bottle tops. It removes all the air from the container, which will extend the shelf life of your juice/smoothie/nut milk and preserve the flavor and appearance for that little bit longer. I make juices in the evening and, next morning, they are basically as good as freshly squeezed.

GARNISHING

Remember to garnish your juices and smoothies. Serve them in beautiful glasses and garnish with fresh berries, fruit, herbs, edible flowers, and other interesting ingredients.

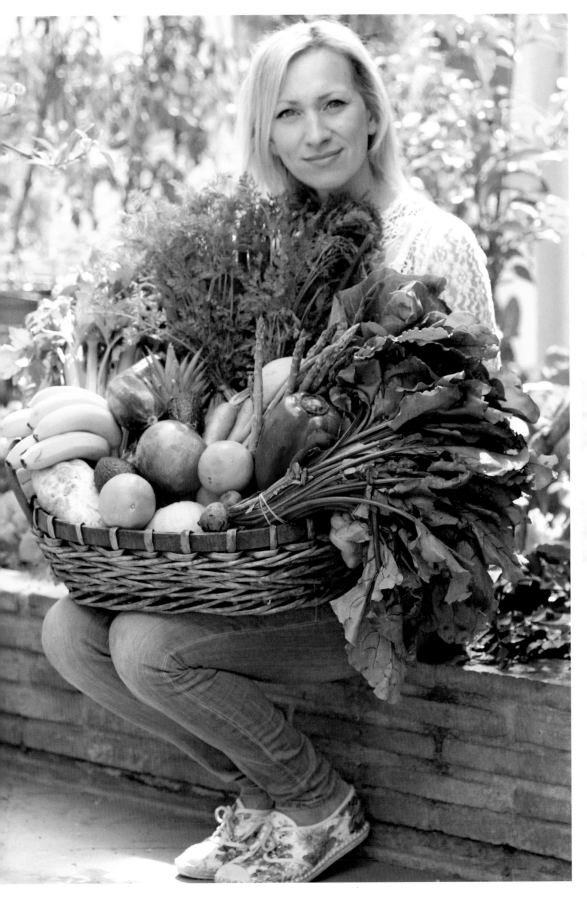

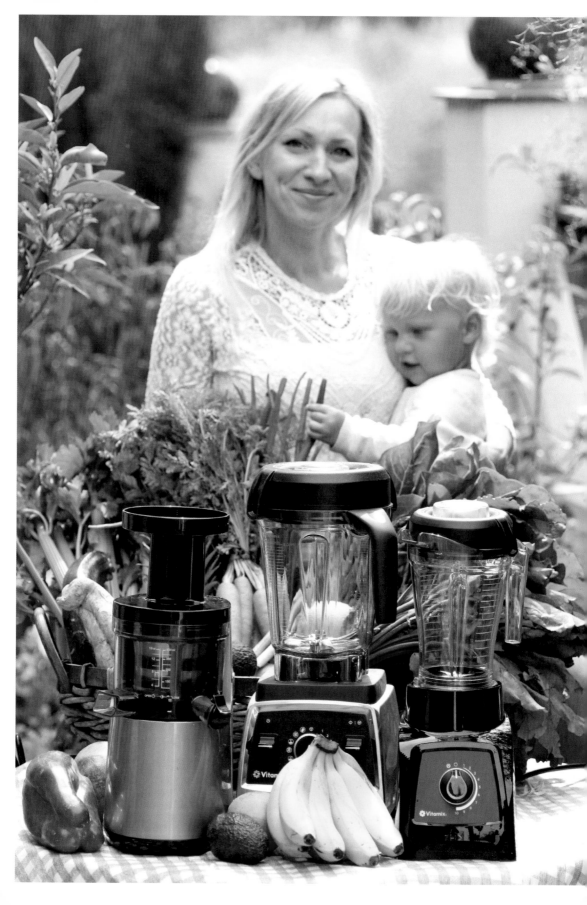

CHOOSING YOUR JUICER AND BLENDER

JUICERS. You need a machine that releases juice in order to make juice from all sorts of vegetables, lettuce, leaves, herbs, and fruit. Juicers come in two main types: centrifugal and slow juicers. Performance and quantities of juice produced vary according to the model you choose. If you plan to juice regularly, it is probably best to invest in a proper slow juicer. But let your budget be your first consideration. Start juicing—you can always upgrade to a better model later on, once freshly squeezed juices become a major part of your lifestyle.

SLOW JUICERS. They crush fruit and vegetables to a fine pulp that is then pressed through a fine metal mesh filter. Slow juicers are slightly more expensive than centrifugal juicers, but they yield considerably more juice. They operate at a much lower speed, which means that they are quieter, that vegetables are juiced more gently, and that the juice does not oxidize as quickly. A juice made with a slow juicer is more nutritious than one made with a centrifugal juicer, because more enzymes are preserved in the process. A juice made with a slow juicer should be consumed within 48 hours or, ideally, straightaway. Wash the juicer immediately after use in order to ensure that no residual fruit flesh dries out and gets stuck to the parts. I have a OMEGA, the easiest-to-clean juicer I have ever owned.

CENTRIFUGAL JUICERS. They shred fruit and vegetables, spinning the pulp through a fine mesh filter. Usually less expensive than slow juicers, they yield less juice. Heat from the rotating blade destroys some of the enzymes, and the juice should be consumed within 24 hours, or ideally straightaway, because the spinning action introduces oxygen, oxidizing the juice and shortening its shelf life. It is important to wash the juicer parts immediately after use to avoid the flesh of fruit and vegetables drying and sticking to them.

BLENDERS. Blenders are a must if you want to make smoothies. Combine all the ingredients in a blender, press the button, and your smoothie is ready to be served.

There are several things to consider when choosing a blender, e.g. the strength of the motor, the number of speed levels, its capacity, and whether or not it crushes ice. If you choose a standard blender in the lower price range, I would recommend one with a glass jar. It is easier to clean and it does not scratch or discolor as easily as those with a plastic jar. Today, jars made of high-quality break-resistant plastic are also available. They do not scratch or discolor either, but they are usually more expensive. A blender does not need to be able to crush ice, but that is certainly an advantage.

If you are making a choice between several different types, bear in mind also how often and how many smoothies you want to make. It pays to invest in a high-quality blender that costs more, lasts longer, has an extended guarantee, and can basically blend any ingredient. A good mixer will chew the ingredients thoroughly, making it easier for the body to absorb the nutrients. I use a Vitamix, which is capable of blending everything from seeds, nuts, ice, frozen fruits, and berries to hard-skinned vegetables.

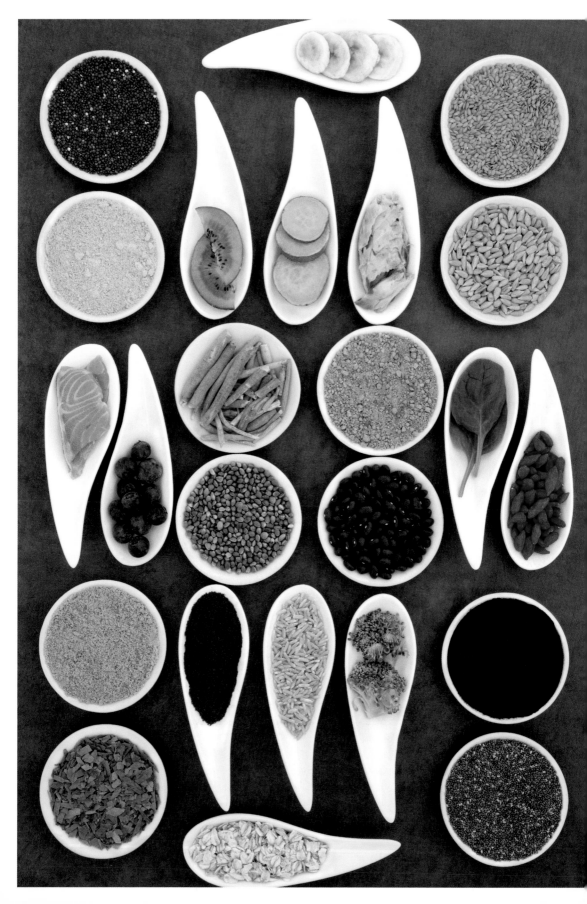

BOOSTING YOUR JUICE OR SMOOTHIE

BERRY POWDERS

If you cannot get hold of fresh berries, berry powders make a good alternative. They are made of whole, freeze-dried berries ground to powder form, including all the pulp, skin, and seeds. Among the many berry powders available, there are those made from açaí, lucuma, maqui, sea buckthorn, blueberry, pome-granate, raspberry, strawberry, rosehip, and cranberry. Berry powders are extremely convenient because they can last for up to 18 months. You can add the powder direct to your juice or smoothie, but be aware that berry flavors are quite concentrated. There are many different varieties you can buy in health food shops. Where possible, choose the organic ones.

SUPERFOODS AND SUPERBERRIES

ACAÍ. Acaí is a superberry native to South American forests and is packed full of antioxidants, vitamins, and essential fats. It contains high levels of vitamin B, vitamin C, minerals, fiber, and protein. Since the berries quickly go off, they are usually sold as pasteurized juice. Unfortunately, pasteurization depletes much of the nutrient content, so freeze-dried acaí powder is a better alternative. The powder can be purchased at any good health food store.

BARLEY GRASS. Barley grass is packed full of vitamins, minerals, amino acids, antioxidants, fiber, and chlo-rophyll. It contains 11 times more calcium and 30 times more vitamin B1 than cow's milk, 5 times more iron than spinach, 7 times more vitamin C than an orange, and 25 times more potassium than a banana. It also contains significant levels of vitamin B12 and 18 different amino acids. Add barley grass powder to your favorite smoothie and drink it on an empty stomach; that way the nutrients will be absorbed more quickly. Store the powder in a dry and cool place, away from direct sunlight. The recommended daily dose is one teaspoon. Barley grass powder is available in health food stores.

CACAO NIBS, RAW. One hundred percent raw, lightly roasted, and crushed cacao nibs. They contain more than three hundred nutrients, including high levels of antioxidants, magnesium, iron, chromium, and vita-min C, as well as serotonin, which makes us happy and content. The fact that cacao is raw means that it has been roasted below 104 °F (40 °C) in order to preserve the beneficial nutrients. They contain no sugar, dairy products, or other additives. Stored airtight, in a cool and dark place, they will keep for a couple of years.

CACAO POWDER, RAW. Raw cacao powder contains more than 300 nutrients, including high levels of antioxidants, magnesium, iron, chromium, vitamin C, and endorphins. The powder is produced by cold-pressing cacao beans and straining off the cacao butter. The temperature is monitored closely during the process—it must not reach above 104 °F (40 °C) in order to ensure no nutrients are lost. The dry cacao expeller cake is ground and then sifted to obtain a fine powder. Cacao powder can easily be combined with other ingredients and is readily absorbed by the body.

You must not confuse raw cacao with regular cocoa or instant chocolate powder. Raw, organic cacao powder is 100 percent cacao that has not been exposed to high temperatures, which is how many nutrients can be lost. Store cacao powder in a cool, dry place, and away from direct sunlight. Unopened, a package will keep for up to a couple of years.

CAMU CAMU. Camu camu is one of the most vitamin C-rich berries around. It contains up to 60 times the amount of the antioxidant vitamin C found in an orange. The berry also contains niacin, thiamin, and riboflavin (B vitamins) as well as the minerals iron, phosphorus, potassium, and calcium. Camu camu is a health bomb, protecting you from free radicals. It can prevent cancer, diabetes, and neurological diseases as well as premature aging. Organic camu camu powder is produced from pitted and dried berries that have gently been milled at low temperatures—all in an effort to optimally preserve the berry's nutrients. The recommended daily dose is ½–1 teaspoon.

GOJI BERRY. The goji berry is a superberry that has a major impact on immunity and that contains 18 different amino acids, 7 of which are essential. The berry also contains essential minerals, such as iron, calcium, zinc, selenium, copper, calcium, germanium, and phosphorus, as well as vitamins B1, B2, B6, and E. Its flavor is a mixture of lingonberries and raisins. The recommended daily dose is ¾–1 ounce (20–30 g) of whole berries (roughly a small handful) or 1 teaspoon of goji berry powder. It should be stored in a cool, dry, and dark place in a sealed container, away from direct sunlight. Once opened, a package of goji berries should be consumed within a couple of months.

INCA BERRY. The inca berry is related to physalis and is as much as 16 percent protein. Inca berries are highly nutritious and contain, among other nutrients, bioflavonoids, which increase cellular uptake of vitamin C. Inca berries also contain phosphorus and vitamins A, C, B1, B2, B6, and B12, as well as plenty of carotenoids and pectin. Pectin is particularly beneficial for digestion and for lowering cholesterol. Dried inca berries are available in well-stocked health food shops.

LUCUMA, POWDER. Lucuma is a nutritious toffee-flavored fruit. It is rich in fiber, antioxidants, vitamins, and minerals—especially vitamins C and B, beta-carotene, calcium, phosphorus, and iron. Lucuma powder contains all of the fruit's nutrients preserved in concentrated form. The powder can be purchased at any good health food store.

MACA ROOT, POWDER. The maca root contains large amounts of amino acids, carbohydrates, and minerals such as calcium, zinc, magnesium, and iron. The maca root also contains vitamins B1, B2, B12, C, and E. Given its rather special flavor, which easily becomes overbearing (it is somewhat reminiscent of horseradish), it is safest to take a little at a time and gradually increase the amount. Mix maca root powder with other bold flavors. It is available in powdered form in health food stores.

MAQUI. The maqui berry contains four times as many antioxidants as the blueberry and twice as many as açaí. This makes maqui an effective weapon against free radicals. In addition, maqui protects the body's cells against oxidative stress and prevents premature aging. Maqui is also bursting with flavonoids, polyphenols, and vitamins A, C, and E, as well as the minerals calcium, potassium, and iron. Freeze-dried maqui powder can be purchased at any good health food store.

MULBERRY. The mulberry contains a lot of vitamin C, vitamin K, iron, and calcium. The mulberry is also a good source of resveratrol, an antioxidant and anti-coagulant substance with a number of beneficial health effects. Dried mulberries can be found in most well-stocked grocery and health food stores. Buy organic berries, if possible. The recommended daily dose is ¾–1 ounce (20–30 g).

ROSEHIP POWDER, WHOLE. Made from whole rosehip berries, i.e. skin, pulp, and seeds. Whole rosehip powder contains 60 times more vitamin C than citrus fruit and is rich in antioxidants and essential minerals, such as iron, calcium, potassium, and magnesium. One tablespoon of whole rosehip powder is equivalent to an entire bowl of fresh rosehips. The recommended daily dose is 1–3 tablespoons, taken with cold drinks or foods. The powder should not be heated above 104 °F (40 °C), as at that temperature the antioxidant effect diminishes. Do not confuse whole rosehip powder with "regular" rosehip soup powder, which contains only the outer layer of the rosehip, as well as sugar and additives. Stored in a dry and cool place, in a sealed package, whole rosehip powder will keep for around a couple of years. People using blood-thinning medication should consult their doctor before starting to take whole rosehip powder.

SEA BUCKTHORN. It is said that a single small sea buckthorn berry contains as much vitamin C as a whole orange. However, the vitamin C content of sea buckthorn varies between 100 and 1,300 milligrams, per 100 grams berries, depending on the variety and ripeness. Sea buckthorn contains vitamin B12, which is very rare in the plant kingdom and which is vital for vegetarians, and it also contains vitamins B1, B2, B3 (niacin), B6, B9 (folic acid), pantothenic acid, biotin, and vitamins E and K.

STINGING NETTLE. Stinging nettle contains plenty of chlorophyll, but also beta-carotene (a provitamin A), calcium, potassium, magnesium, iron, silicon, manganese, flavonoids, vitamins C, B, and K, as well as folic acid. The stinging effect disappears when nettle is dried or boiled. Pick young shoots and dry, blanche, or freeze them. Nettle is also available in powder form. Dried nettles should be stored in a dark place, in a sealed container, and can last for around two years.

WHEATGRASS. Containing more than 20 amino acids, several hundred enzymes, 90 minerals, and a whole lot of vitamins, wheatgrass is an almost complete food. It is around 70 percent chlorophyll, which is not only the building block of the plant kingdom but also beneficial for humans. Add wheatgrass powder to your favorite smoothie and drink it on an empty stomach; that way the nutrients will be absorbed more quickly. Store it in a dry and cool place, away from direct sunlight. The recommended daily dose is one teaspoon. Wheatgrass powder is available in health food stores.

ALGAE

Algae are a very good source of protein. The body can absorb four times more protein from the blue-green alga spirulina than from meat. Spirulina is sometimes spoken of as the alga that can solve world hunger. It contains so many nutrients that NASA usually instructs its astronauts to take spirulina with them on space flights. Other beneficial algae include chlorella, arame, wakame, and dulse.

CHLORELLA. Chlorella is a unicellular green alga that has existed on Earth for several hundred million years. It is around 60 percent protein and contains a large number of important amino acids. Chlorella also contains essential vitamins and minerals, such as vitamins A, C, and E, and several B vitamins, as well as iron, calcium, and magnesium. It is also rich in chlorophyll, which helps to boost the immune system and cleanse the blood. Chlorella is considered to cleanse the body of heavy metals and other toxins, improve digestion, and neutralize the body's pH value, which is usually too acidic.

SPIRULINA. Spirulina is an extremely nutritious alga that is largely made up of protein, but it also contains essential minerals, vitamins, fatty acids, and antioxidants. Spirulina is also considered to improve the immune system, prevent harmful bacterial and viral growth, and have a protective effect against cancer. Spirulina can also improve memory and learning ability, and prevent and relieve hay fever. The recommended daily dose is 1 teaspoon. Spirulina should be stored in a dry and cool place.

PROTEIN POWDERS

Examples of good vegan protein powders are raw rice protein, pea protein, hemp protein, oat protein, tempeh, miso, ground nuts, soy milk, and algae. For example, spirulina is up to 65 percent protein. Ask for more information and advice in your health food store.

BENEFICIAL OILS

It is fine to use beneficial cold-pressed oils in your smoothies. Examples include coconut oil, flaxseed oil, and hempseed oil. Ask for more information and advice in your health food store.

COCONUT OIL. Coconut oil is one of the world's healthiest oils. It is solid at room temperature but turns liquid at around 75 °F (24 °C). Some 50 percent of the lipids in coconut oil consist of lauric acid, which the body converts to monolaurin acid, which is antiviral, antifungal, and antibacterial. Coconut oil is as suitable for cooking, smoothies, and desserts as it is for body care. Always buy organic, raw, cold-pressed, unbleached, unrefined, and deodorized coconut oil. The list of ingredients should read 100 percent coconut. It should be stored in a cool and dark place. Coconut oil is available in grocery and health food stores.

FLAXSEED OIL. Flaxseed oil is produced from cold-pressed flax seeds and, depending on the brand, contains 50–65 percent omega-3 fatty acids. Other ingredients include omega-6 and omega-9 fatty acids, and vitamin E. Ideally, buy organic and cold-pressed flaxseed oil. The recommended daily dose is 1–2 teaspoons. Store your opened bottle of flaxseed oil in the fridge and use it within 4 weeks. It is available in health food stores.

HEMPSEED OIL. Hempseed oil is produced by pressing hemp seeds. Hempseed oil is considered one of nature's most beneficial vegetable oils because it contains the highest levels of polyunsaturated fatty acids. Organic, cold-pressed hempseed oil is an excellent food for vegetarians and vegans because it ensures a balanced protein intake. In addition, hempseed oil contains a lot of omega-3, omega-6, and omega-9 fatty acids, which are otherwise obtained from fish. Store your opened bottle of hempseed oil in the fridge and use it within 4 weeks. It is available in health food stores.

NUT BUTTERS

Nut butters have become popular with health-conscious people thanks to their high fiber content, protein, healthy fats, minerals, vitamins, and antioxidants. They also have a satiating effect. A high-quality nut butter should be organically produced and contain at least 99 percent nuts. It should not contain anything else except, possibly, a little sea salt. However, if you want to add a nut butter to your smoothies, it is best to use unsalted. There are many different types of nut butter out there, but unfortunately some of them contain both palm oil and sugar—so do watch out for these ingredients! Add nut butter direct to your smoothie, or make nut milk by blending some butter with water only. Nut butters are available in health food stores and well-stocked grocery stores.

NUTS AND SEEDS

During a detox, it is important that you have light snacks so you can keep your spirits up and not get too hungry. A handful of nuts and seeds is a perfect snack. Remember always to buy natural, unroasted, preferably organic, nuts and seeds. Most nuts should be soaked overnight in order to disable hard-to-digest enzymes. You can make tasty nut milk from nuts: for details see page 37.

ALMONDS. Sweet almonds contain a lot of beneficial monounsaturated fat as well as plenty of protein and vitamin E. To boost your smoothie, add some organic almond butter, which you can buy in health food stores.

BRAZIL NUTS. In addition to lots of protein, Brazil nuts contain selenium and zinc. Brazil nuts are 70 percent fat, the bulk of which is omega-6 fatty acids and the smaller part omega-3 fatty acids. Brazil nuts should be white inside; a yellow tinge means that the fats have started to go rancid.

HAZELNUTS. Hazelnuts contain high levels of vitamin E and protein, as well as some fat.

HEMP SEEDS. Hemp seeds contain high levels of both beneficial polyunsaturated fatty acids and omega-3 and omega-6. The seeds are as much as 25 percent protein and are rich in essential amino acids. They also contain high levels of calcium, magnesium, phosphorus, sulfur, carotene, iron, and zinc as well as vitamins C, E, B1, B2, B3, and B6. Hemp seeds come in several different forms: shelled, unshelled, or as hemp protein powder, which is excellent as a natural protein supplement.

PECANS. Pecans are 72 percent fat, 63 percent of which is unsaturated. They also contain high levels of antioxidants. Much of their nutrient content is found in the brown inner shell.

PINE NUTS. Pine nuts contain a lot of zinc, iron, protein, and unsaturated fat.

PISTACHIOS. Pistachios contain a lot of fat and protein. Strictly speaking, they are actually seeds, not nuts, and can therefore usually be consumed by people with nut allergies.

PUMPKIN SEEDS. Pumpkin seeds contain zinc and antioxidants among other ingredients. They are high in protein and contain a lot of unsaturated fat. Pumpkin seeds are also anti-inflammatory and strengthen immunity.

SESAME SEEDS. Sesame seeds are 50 percent fat, almost all of which is beneficial. They are also high in protein—18 percent. Ground sesame seeds are a delicious addition to your smoothies and are available in health food stores.

SUNFLOWER SEEDS. Sunflower seeds are obtained from the center of the sunflower head. They are rich in vitamin E, omega-6, and monounsaturated fatty acids. The also contain vitamin B5, which is believed to help the body to cope with stress.

WALNUTS. Walnuts are extremely healthful, especially for vegetarians, because they contain large amounts of omega-3.

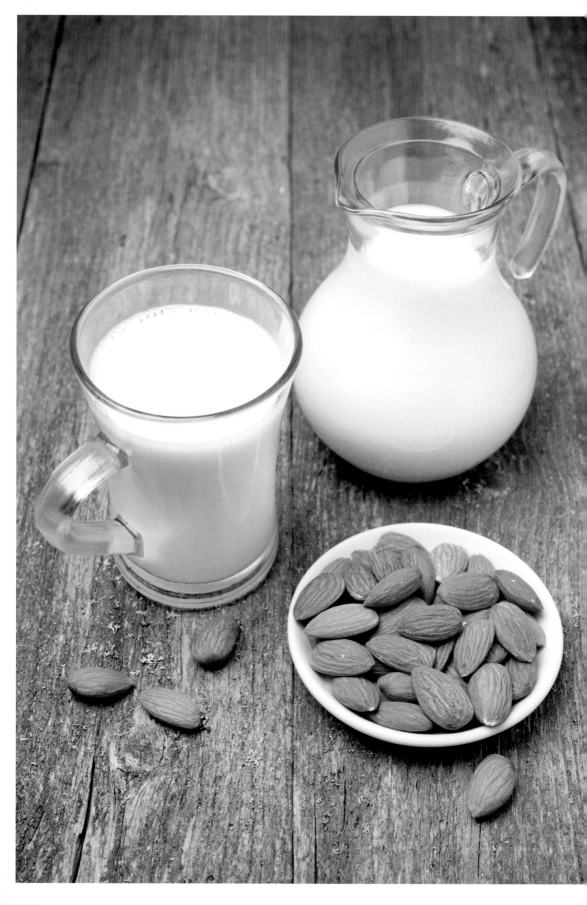

NUT, SEED, AND OAT MILK

Making your own nut milk is easy. In addition to tasting good, it is a healthy alternative to regular milk, which you should avoid during a detox, and an excellent replacement if you are lactose-intolerant or vegan.

Milk can be made from a variety of nuts and seeds, e.g. hemp seeds, cashews, hazelnuts, pumpkin seeds, pecans, pistachios, walnuts, sunflower seeds, and almonds. Choose unsalted, unroasted, and organic nuts and seeds—they deliver most on taste, contain the highest nutrient levels, and are free from pesticides and other "nasties."

Soak your nuts overnight in a cool place in order to eliminate hard-to-digest enzymes and make the flavor milder. Hazelnuts need no pre-soaking as they do not contain enzyme inhibitors. You can even make milk from coconut flakes and shelled hemp seeds in a blender.

Strain off the soaking water and rinse the nuts properly. Add some fresh water and blend until the nuts become homogenized in the liquid. Strain the milk using a nut-milk bag or a fine-mesh sieve (shelled hemp seeds do not need to be strained!) and squeeze out as much of the liquid as possible. Season with pure vanilla, cinnamon, cardamom, or raw cacao and sweeten to taste with organic figs, apricots, medjool dates, or organic honey.

Store the milk in a glass bottle or jar—that way it will keep longer than in a plastic container, 3–5 days in the refrigerator. Nut milk can also easily be frozen in ice-cube trays. The leftover nut pulp can be used to make nut balls, muesli, or bread, or it can be stirred into your morning porridge.

ALMOND, NUT, AND SEED MILK
1 cup (140 g) soaked nuts, seeds, or almonds + 4 cups (1 liter) water + 1 pinch Himalayan salt.

OAT MILK
1 cup (90 g) soaked organic oatmeal + 4 cups (1 liter) water + 1 pinch Himalayan salt.

SESAME MILK
1 cup (130 g) soaked sesame seeds + 4 cups (1 liter) water + 1 pinch Himalayan salt.

SOY MILK
1 cup (175 g) soaked soybeans or ¾ cup soybean meal + 4 cups (1 liter) water + 1 pinch Himalayan salt.

COCONUT MILK
1 cup (90 g) raw, shredded coconut + 4 cups (1 liter) water + 1 pinch Himalayan salt.

HEMP MILK
¾ cup (120 g) shelled hemp seeds + 4 cups (1 liter) water + 1 pinch Himalayan salt.

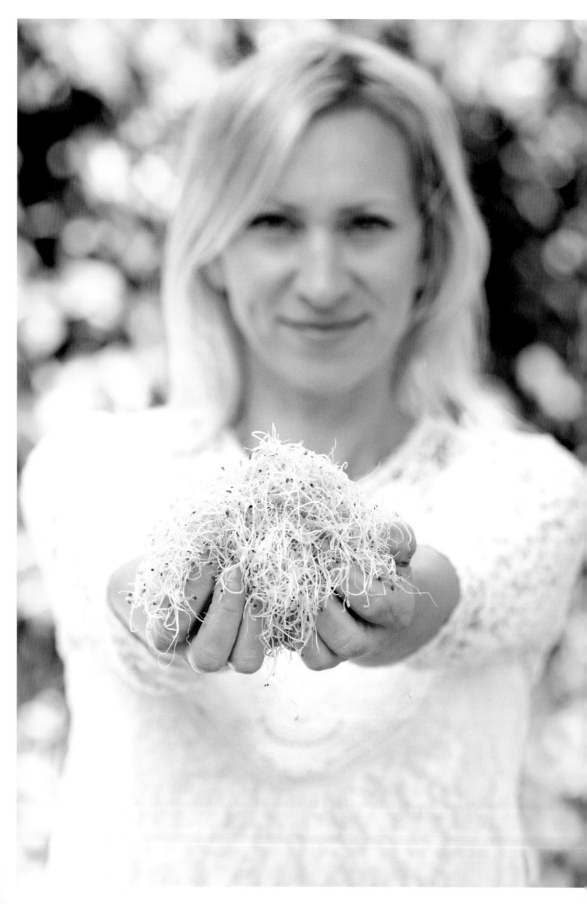

ON SPROUTS AND SPROUTING AT HOME

Chockfull of nutrients and enzymes, sprouts make a tasty and beneficial addition to your diet. You can benefit from growing your own organic sprouts at home all year round—simple, inexpensive, and always available.

A sprout is the beginning of life and contains valuable substances, such as vegetable protein, unsaturated fatty acids, and essential minerals. When a seed sprouts, its essential vitamin B and E content increases enormously. We are most in need of these vitamins after winter, in order to strengthen our immunity and fend off spring fatigue.

There are many different varieties of seeds around. In principle, any seed can be sprouted. Seeds for sprouting are available online or in health food stores. On the back of the seed packet you will find instructions on how to grow your seeds. The method varies depending on the seed variety. Some take a longer time to sprout, some are sprouted in the dark, while others need soil to grow.

The seeds you can use for sprouting include: alfalfa, amaranth, barley berries, buckwheat, clover, corn, cress, fenugreek, millet, mung beans, oats, pumpkin, quinoa, radish, raw rice, rye, sesame, spelt, sunflower seeds, wheat berries, and various types of lentils.

There are various sprouting methods if you want to sprout at home. For example, you can use a simple glass jar. Attach a clean piece of straining cloth over the mouth of the jar; this works not only to aerate the sprouts but also to sieve them when you need to change the water. You can also buy a sprouting jar with a mesh screen lid. Special sprouters (germinators) or multi-tiered plastic trays can be used to sprout different types of sprouts at the same time. I use one from BioSnacky. Also available are easy-to-use sprouting nets or bags. There is a special machine that makes the whole process easier and uses it to full effect, but it is an expensive option and one you probably will not need when starting out. A cheaper, homemade option (described above) will work just as well and adds more to the simplistic charm of sprouts grown inexpensively at home. Place the jar with the rinsed seeds or sprouts in a place that is not too light or cool.

Sprout = the plant's embryo, i.e. the first stage of growth. Sprouts are usually white or light green in color. They are mini threads with the seed attached to one end.

Shoot = a seed that has sprouted and then developed into a small, short, bright stalk, usually with small green leaves at the top.

Any problems? You may notice from time to time that your sprouts have developed an off smell and that they feel warm to the touch. This is usually due to the fact that you have crammed too many seeds into the jar and so no air can come in. There are some seeds that are old and others that are inherently poor germinators; neither will work. Your sprouts can also go off if you forget to rinse them. If this is the case, throw out your seeds or sprouts, rinse out the jar, and start a new batch. Be sure to rinse and store the sprouts according to directions. Sprouts are a sensitive, perishable food and have a short shelf life. They easily ferment and become moldy. Always check the freshness and purchase date.

Use. Sprouts can be added to smoothies or eaten as they are. Or, if they have developed to a full-fledged grass stage, you can juice them as well. Sprouts and shoots are usually used as a filling for sandwiches or are tossed into salads. They can also be used in soups, stews, wok-type dishes, sauces, etc., in which case they should be added to the dish as late as possible to preserve their form, flavor, and vitamin content.

Shelf life and storage. A convenient way to store ready-to-eat sprouts is in the refrigerator because the cold will stop the sprouting process. Sprouts have a short shelf life: 3–4 days at most. It is best to eat them freshly harvested. Rinse them every day and before use. Shoots have a longer shelf life than sprouts: around one week.

Points to remember when sprouting
» Keep the seeds moist.
» Seeds that are too moist can become moldy.
» Do not pick and poke sprouts with your fingers: use a spoon instead.
» Rinse twice a day.
» Clean the sprouting jar before starting a new batch.
» Sprouts should be stored in a dark place before they are ready to eat.
» Sometimes you will notice a white film, but do not confuse it with mold. If you rinse the sprouts, it will disappear.

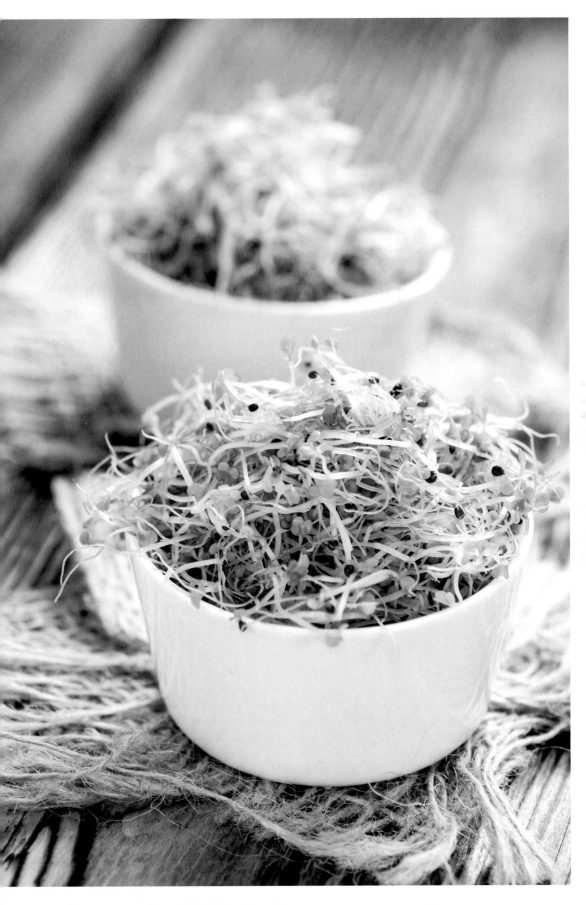

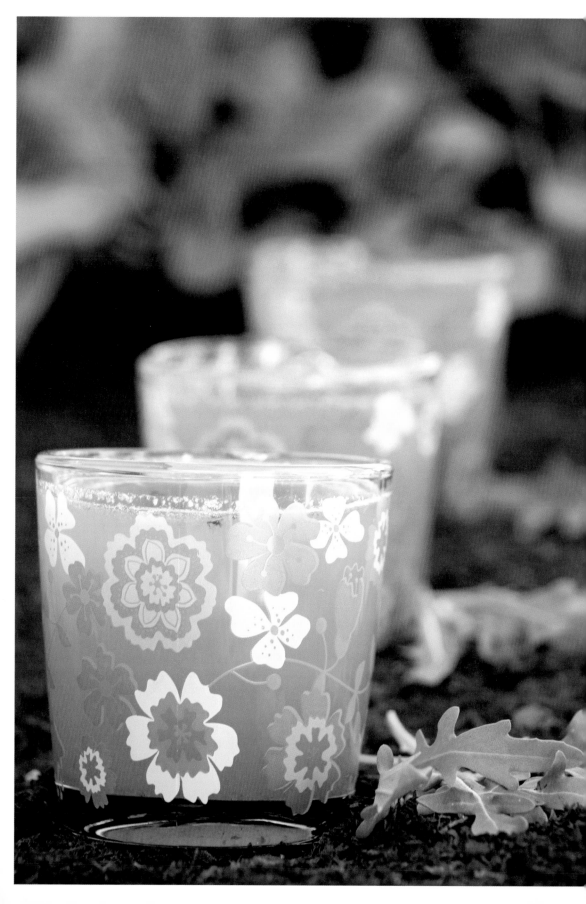

SPICY ARUGULA JUICE

Arugula is high in vitamins A, C, and K and is rich in iron and calcium. Arugula also contains lutein, which is good for the eyes and skin. Like basil and parsley, arugula was originally grown as a herb for cooking in the Mediterranean region, but nowadays it is used more as a salad leaf. Arugula is a member of the cabbage family and is related to cauliflower, kale, and broccoli. The small green leaves will keep for around a week in the refrigerator, but only for a day at room temperature.

Makes one glass

Generous ¾ cup / 200 ml coconut water

2 handfuls (approx. 2½ oz / 70 g) arugula

1 bunch (approx. ¾ oz / 20 g) cilantro

½–1 red chili pepper (according to taste)

2 green apples

Rinse the ingredients. Pour the coconut water into a large glass. Cut the apples into wedges and juice together with the arugula, cilantro, and chili pepper. Pour the juice into the glass with the coconut water, stir, and serve.

RED BEET AND CELERY JUICE

Red beets contain calcium, vitamin C, iron, magnesium, phosphorus, and manganese among other nutrients. Red beets cleanse the blood and promote red blood cell growth. Studies have shown that beets increase the body's capacity to take up oxygen, which improves stamina during exercise. Beets are also considered helpful against high blood pressure and gastric ulcers. They remove toxins from the intestines, liver, and gallbladder.

Makes one glass

½ lemon

1 yellow bell pepper

2 stalks celery

½ cucumber

2 red beets

Rinse the ingredients. Remove the zest of the lemon, taking care not to remove the nutritious white pith beneath. Trim the tops and bottoms of the beets and chop all the ingredients into pieces small enough to feed through the juicer. Juice, pour into a glass, and serve.

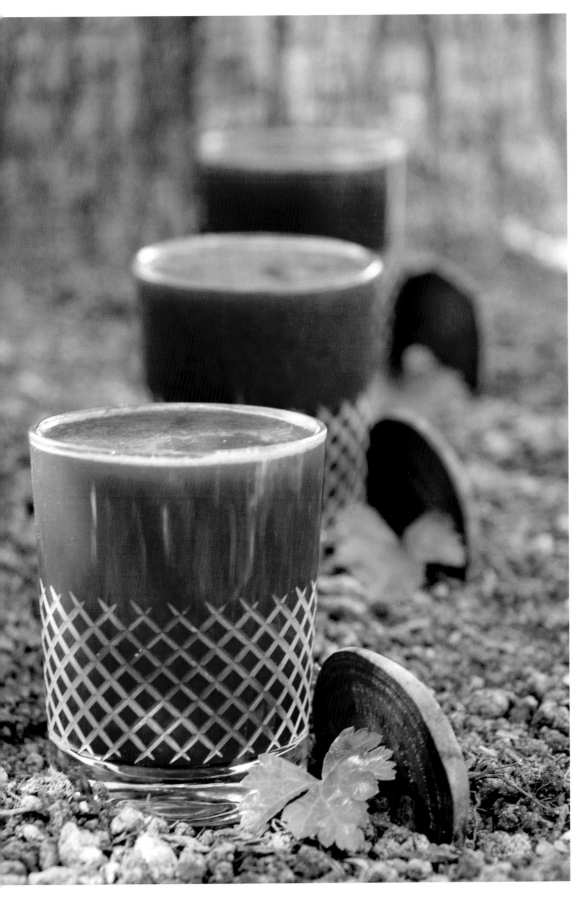

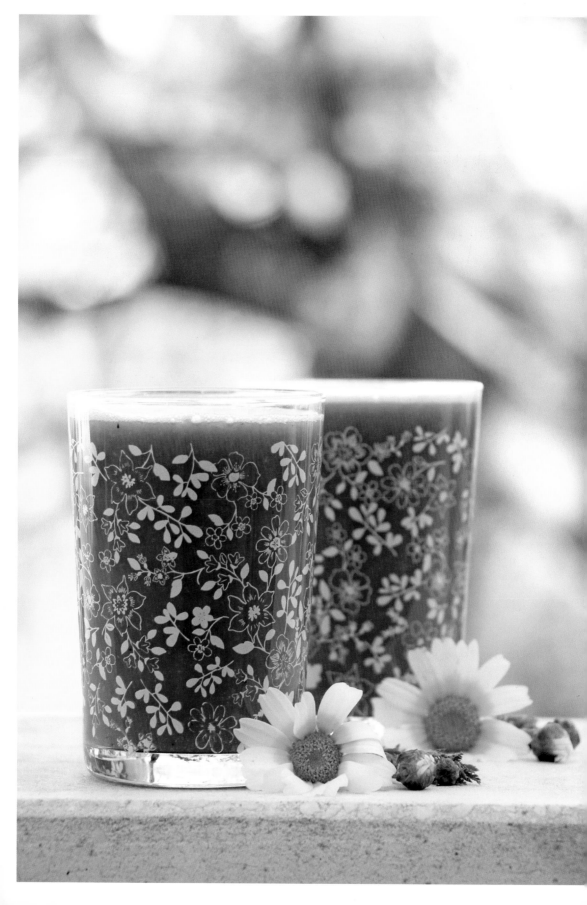

WHEATGRASS AND ORANGE JUICE

Wheatgrass is rich in natural vitamins A and C. In addition to being an unusually good source of vitamin B, it is also an excellent source of calcium, iron, magnesium, phosphorus, potassium, sodium, sulfur, cobalt, zinc, and protein. Wheatgrass juice cleanses the blood. It helps to combat high blood pressure as it reduces the amount of toxins in the body and supplies iron to the blood, thereby improving blood circulation. Wheatgrass contains no gluten.

Growing your own wheatgrass is simple. Soak the wheat berries and allow them to sprout for a day or two, rinsing frequently. Spread a ½–1-inch / 1–2 cm layer of soil on a seed tray, flatten the soil, and moisten it. Place the sprouted wheat berries all over the soil layer without pressing them into the soil. Spray with water to moisten them several times a day during the first three days, and then water as you would a potted plant. Make sure you keep the soil evenly moist. Place the tray in a light spot. The wheatgrass is ready for harvesting when it reaches 7 inches / 18 cm in height. Harvest by cutting off a handful close to the grain.

Makes one glass

2 oranges

2 handfuls wheatgrass

1 handful arugula

1 stalk celery

Rinse the ingredients. Remove the zest of the oranges, taking care not to remove the nutritious white pith beneath. Feed all the ingredients through a juicer. Pour and serve.

LIME AND MINT JUICE

Lime is the tartest of all citrus fruits and brightens up a juice nicely. Like all other citrus fruits, lime contains a lot of vitamin C. Lime juice also has an antibacterial effect and is used in some countries as a cure for acne and cold sores.

Squeezing juice out of a lime can be hard work, but you will get roughly twice as much juice if you roll the lime back and forth on the countertop, firmly pressing down with one hand, before cutting it in two. You can freeze the juice for later use by pouring it into an ice-cube tray and storing the cubes in a plastic freezer bag.

Makes one glass

1 lime

1 handful mint

1 handful spinach

½ cucumber

1 red apple

Rinse the ingredients. Remove the zest of the lime, taking care not to remove the nutritious white pith beneath. Chop all the ingredients into small pieces and feed through the juicer. Pour into a glass and serve with a sprig of mint.

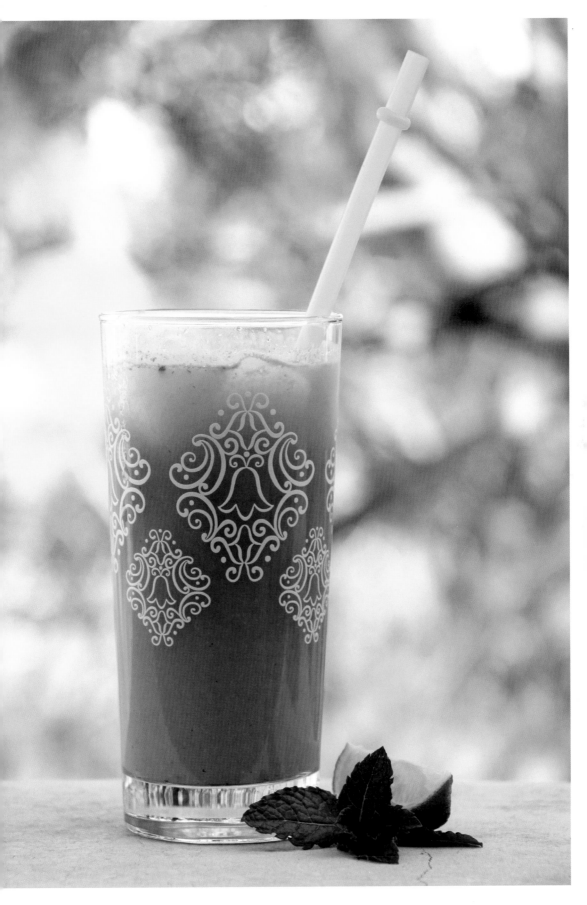

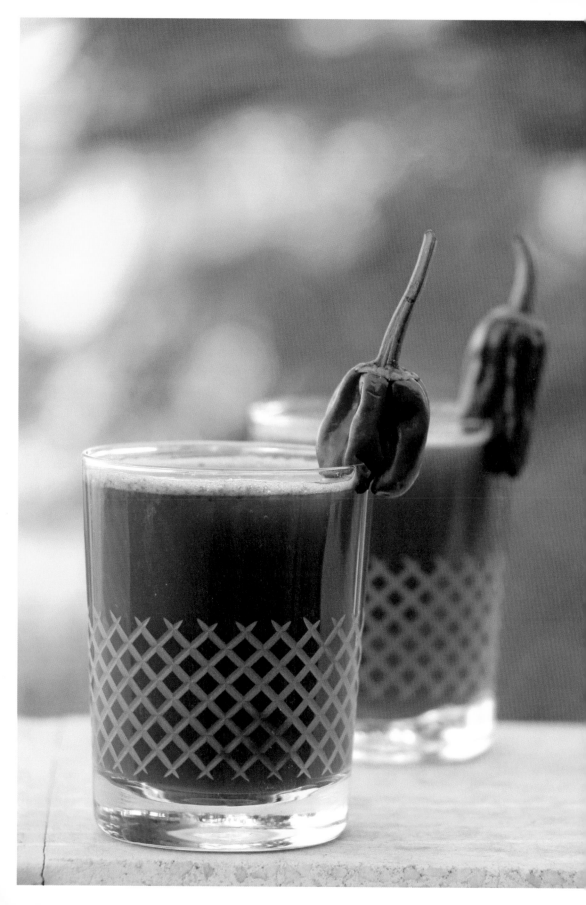

BELL PEPPER AND JALAPEÑO JUICE

Growing your own bell peppers is simple. Save the cores, i.e. the seeds, and leave them to dry on a sheet of kitchen paper for a day or two. Sow a few seeds (approximately ⅕ inch / ½ cm deep) in a jiffy (peat) pot or a pot filled with seed compost, water them, and place a plastic bag over the pot. The plants will begin to appear in around a couple of weeks. Wait for another couple of weeks and then repot each plant in a separate pot filled with potting soil, leaving them in a sunny place indoors. Don't forget to brush the flowers to pollinate them, otherwise you will not get any fruit. This is not necessary if the pots are left outdoors. If you sow the seeds in May, you will have bell peppers as early as August.

Makes one glass

2 green bell peppers

3 jalapeños

½ cucumber

2 handfuls arugula

1 red apple

Rinse the ingredients and chop them into small pieces. Feed all the ingredients through a juicer. Pour into a glass and serve.

GREEN STRAWBERRY AND ORANGE JUICE

Just 1¼ cups / 125 g of strawberries provide the recommended daily amount of vitamin C and a third of the recommended daily amount of folate or folic acid, which is a B vitamin. Strawberries also contain plenty of fiber and minerals such as potassium, iron, and zinc. They are rich in antioxidants.

Makes one glass

1 orange

2 stalks celery

1 handful spinach

½ head romaine lettuce

1 cup / 100 g strawberries

Rinse all the ingredients. Remove the zest of the orange, taking care not to remove the nutritious white pith beneath. Chop the ingredients into smaller pieces and process in a juicer. Pour into a glass and serve.

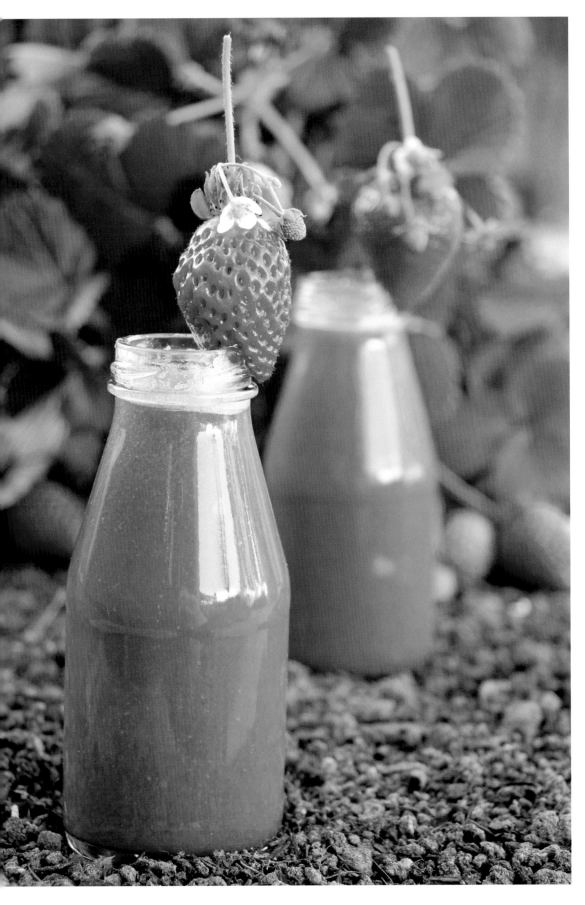

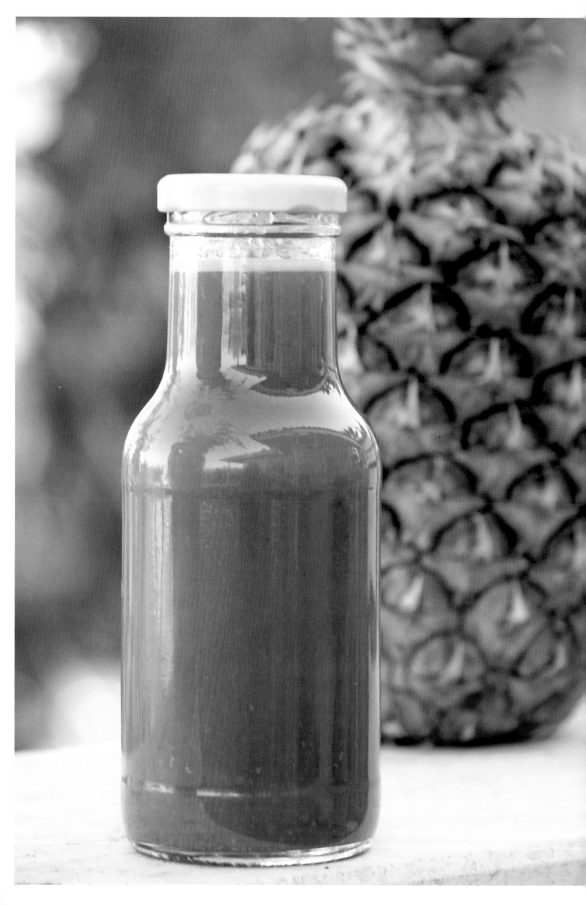

GREEN PINEAPPLE JUICE

Sweet and delicious, pineapple contains high quantities of beneficial fiber and vitamins that protect against viruses and infections. Pineapple is mainly rich in vitamin C, which helps build connective tissue and assists the body in absorbing iron from food. Vitamin C is also an antioxidant, offering protection against free radicals, which have harmful effects on the body's cells. In addition to vitamins, pineapple is rich in bromelain—an extremely potent enzyme that breaks down protein—that, in turn, aids digestion. Bromelain is also good for blood circulation because it decreases blood pressure.

Look out for plump fruit when buying pineapples. To test if a pineapple is ripe, gently pull off one of the leaves. If it comes off easily, the pineapple is ripe. But beware, it may also be overripe, so to be on the safe side, choose one whose leaves don't come off readily and allow it to ripen at home.

Makes one glass

1 lime

½ pineapple

½ head Savoy cabbage

1 handful spinach

1 oz / 25 g fresh ginger

Rinse the ingredients. Remove the zest of the lime, taking care not to remove the nutritious white pith beneath. Remove the leafy crown of the pineapple and cut away the hard skin. Chop all the ingredients into small pieces and feed through a juicer. Pour into a glass and serve.

MELON AND KIWI JUICE

If you wash a kiwi, you can safely eat the skin—and it's beneficial, too. The skin is soft and tasty and it won't feel furry in the mouth. Kiwi contains large amounts of vitamin C, as well as vitamin E. Be careful not to eat kiwi with dairy. It should be combined with other berries and tropical fruit.

Till the 1960s kiwi was commonly known as Chinese gooseberry. New Zealand is a major exporter of kiwis, but the fruit is also available from Mediterranean countries between the months of November and April. A ripe kiwi should yield to gentle pressure. Avoid kiwis that are overripe as they can taste unpleasant.

Makes one glass

½ honeydew melon

2 kiwis

1 stalk celery

1 bunch parsley

½ head broccoli

Rinse the ingredients. Peel the melon, using a vegetable peeler if the skin is hard. Leave the nutritious seeds inside. Chop all the ingredients into small pieces and feed through a juicer. Pour into a glass and serve.

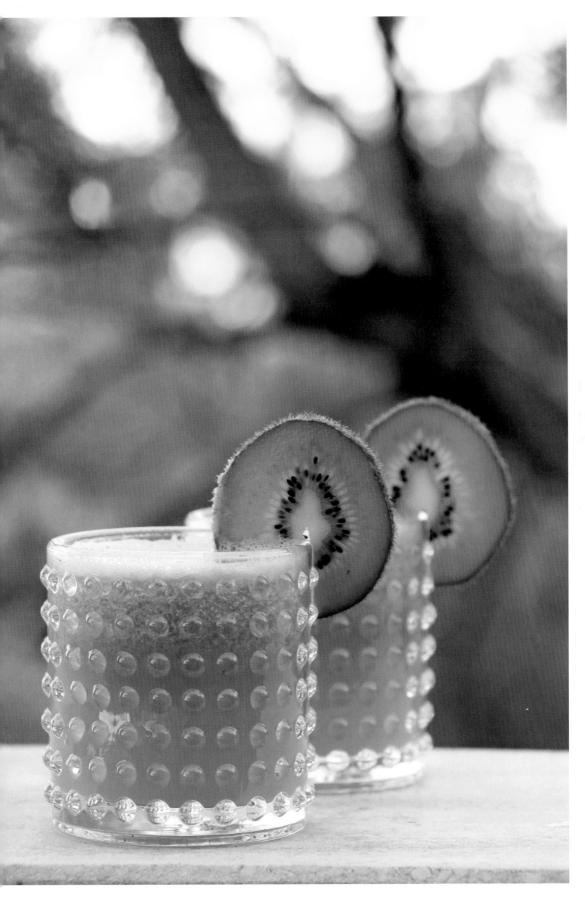

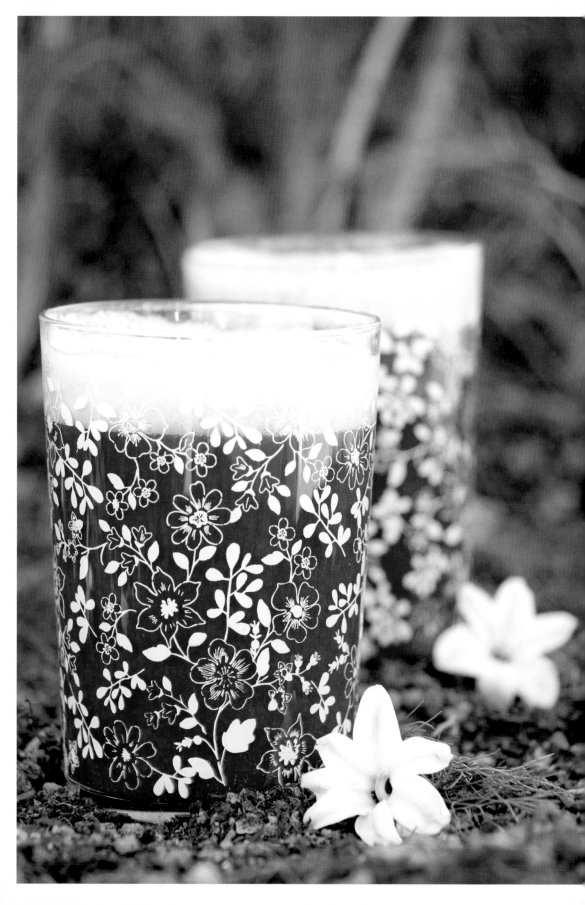

FENNEL AND BLUEBERRY JUICE

Blueberries contain powerful antioxidants and are sometimes called superberries. They are good for the skin, vision, and night vision—and they may help to prevent glaucoma by reducing intraocular pressure. Blueberries are also said to be good for blood circulation in the legs and for combating varicose veins, inflammation, blood clots, high blood pressure, and "bad" LDL cholesterol. The berries are also beneficial to diabetics because they regulate blood sugar. Blueberries can be beneficial in the treatment of urinary tract infections and diarrhea.

Wild blueberries are especially wholesome as they contain abundant amounts of flavonoids, carotene, vitamin C, vitamin B6, and magnesium.

Makes one glass

1 lemon

2 fennels

⅓ head red cabbage

2 red apples

1 cup / 100 g blueberries, frozen

Rinse the ingredients. Remove the zest of the lemon, taking care not to remove the nutritious white pith beneath. Chop the fennel, apples, and red cabbage into small pieces and feed all the ingredients, apart from the blueberries, through a juicer. Pour the juice into a blender and blend in the frozen blueberries. (If you want to wash fewer dishes or extract just the juice from the blueberries without the pulp, run the blueberries through the juicer, but bear in mind that they'll defrost.) Pour into a glass and serve.

SWEET POTATO AND GINGER JUICE

The part of ginger used in cooking or for medicinal purposes is the actual rhizome, which grows horizontally just below the soil surface. Ginger is grown in pretty much the same way as potatoes, by planting the rhizome below ground level. The plant then shoots up above ground, reaching several feet in height and producing blossoms and leaves. Ginger can also be grown at home by planting gingerroots in a pot filled with potting soil. It must never be allowed to dry out. The shoots reach a height of around 3 feet 3 inches / 1 meter. Once established the plant may produce pink blossoms.

Makes one glass

1 sweet potato

2 carrots

½ red beet

1 generous handful wheat-grass

1 oz / 25 g fresh ginger

Rinse the ingredients. Trim the tops of all the root vegetables and chop them into small pieces. Feed all the ingredients through a juicer. Pour into a glass and serve.

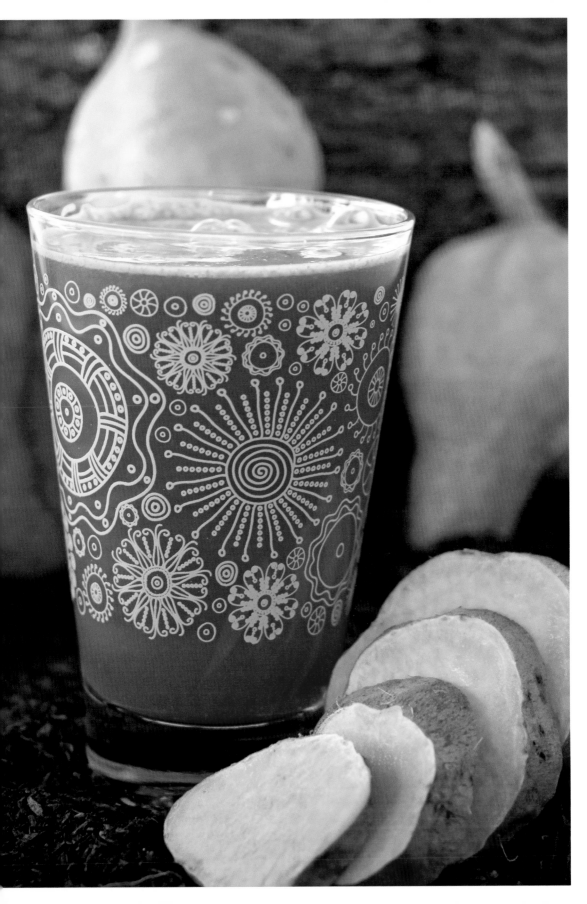

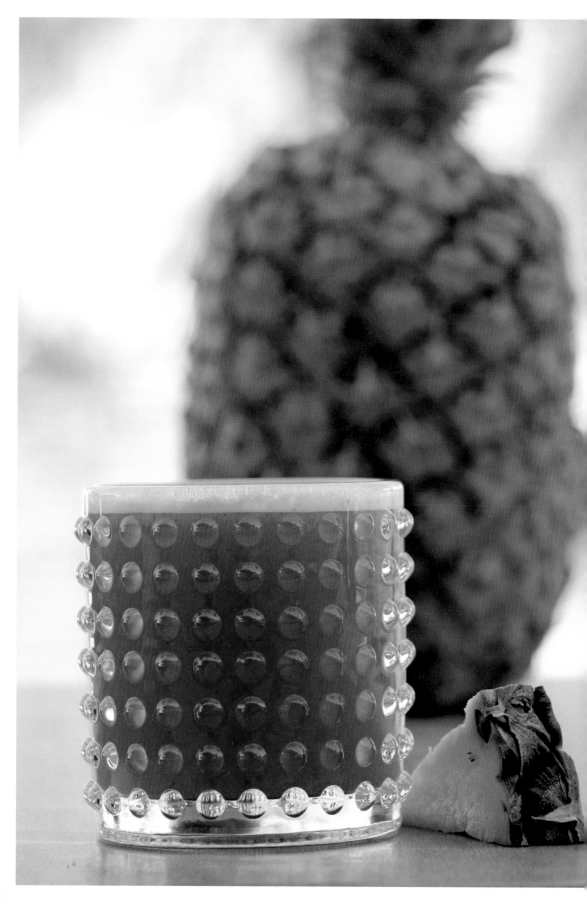

GREEN RASPBERRY AND PINEAPPLE JUICE

Raspberries contain a whole array of beneficial ingredients that keep us healthy and alert. These superberries are anti-inflammatory, they strengthen immunity, and they contain substances that are said to fight cancer and protect against heart disease. Raspberries are rich in fiber, which helps to keep cholesterol levels down. The berries contain a lot of vitamin C, folic acid, iron, calcium, and potassium. Raspberries also have an expectorant and detoxifying effect and can relieve menstrual pain.

Buy raspberries that are uniform in color. The berries go off easily and should be used within a couple of days. Stock up during raspberry season and freeze. Health food stores sell freeze-dried raspberry powder, which also works really well in smoothies.

Makes one glass

1 cup / 100 g raspberries, fresh or defrosted

2 handfuls spinach

½ pineapple

Rinse the ingredients. Remove the leafy crown of the pineapple, cut away the hard skin, and chop the flesh into small pieces. Feed all the ingredients through a juicer. Pour into a glass and serve.

If you want to use the pulp in the smoothie, blend all the ingredients in a blender instead and dilute with a little water.

KALE AND GINGER JUICE

Kale is called "the Queen of Greens" because it has the highest vitamin content of all the brassicas (broccoli, cauliflower, white cabbage, red cabbage, and Brussels sprouts). Kale is rich in vitamins C, A, K, and B6 and also contains calcium, iron, copper, manganese, phosphorus, potassium, and several other minerals. Like all brassicas, kale promotes good intestinal bacteria, cleanses the blood, and detoxifies the body. Kale is also reported to contain cancer-fighting substances—it and other brassicas may have the ability to limit cell growth in pancreatic cancer and reduce the risk of lung, gallbladder, urinary bladder, prostate, ovarian, and colon cancer.

The great thing about kale is that it is available from October to March, at a time of year when there are not so many other vegetables that are grown locally or naturally.

Makes one glass

8 leaves kale

3 carrots

½ lemon

½ cucumber

2 oz / 50 g fresh ginger

Rinse all the ingredients, chop them into small pieces, and feed through a juicer. Pour into a glass and serve.

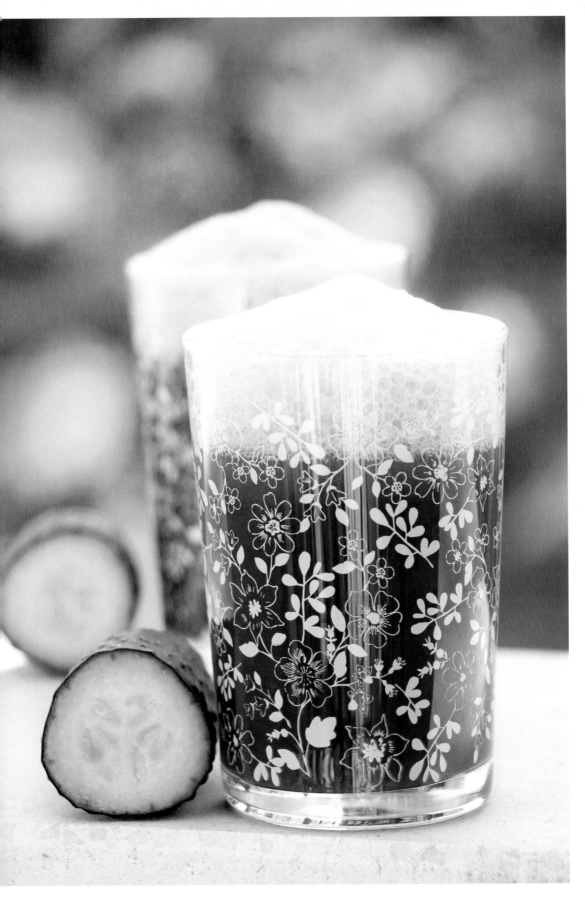

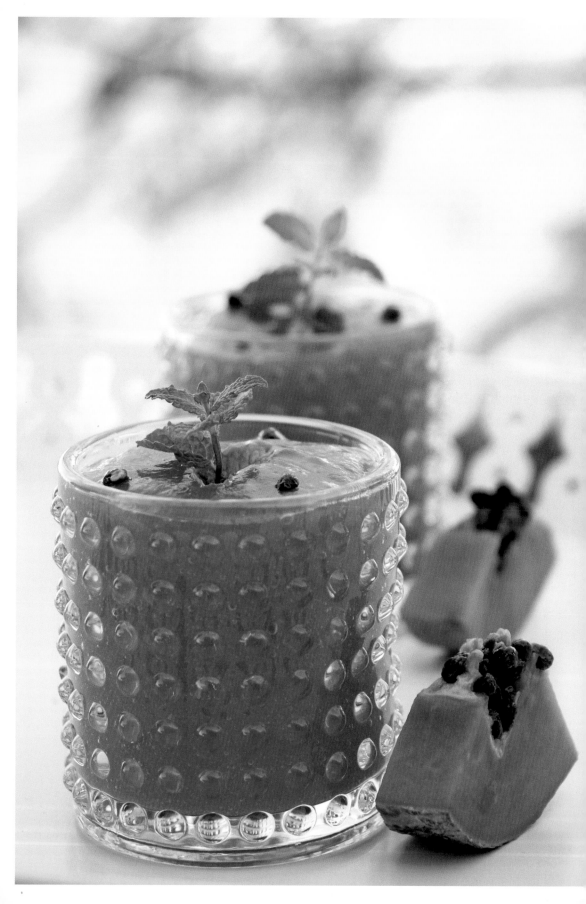

PAPAYA AND MINT JUICE

Papaya is rich in vitamins A, C, E, and B as well as containing high amounts of several antioxidants, such as carotene, zeaxanthin, and flavonoids. It also contains several essential minerals, such as potassium, magnesium, calcium, and iron. Papaya contains the enzyme papain, which is used in treatments for indigestion. Papaya is also said to be effective in weight loss.

Makes one glass

1 lime

1 medium-size papaya, skin on and seeds in

1 bunch mint

Rinse the ingredients. Remove the zest of the lime, taking care not to remove the nutritious white pith beneath. You do not have to peel the papaya, and you can leave the seeds in if you want—they are nutritious but taste peppery. Chop the papaya into small pieces and feed all the ingredients through a juicer. Pour into a glass and serve.

FENNEL AND TOMATO JUICE

Fennel is a member of the same vegetable family as carrot, dill, and parsley. In general, you can eat all parts of a fennel plant—root, stem, leaves, and seeds. Fennel is rich in vitamins A, B, and C as well as fiber, sodium, iron, zinc, and essential oils.

Fennel keeps for a couple of days at room temperature, or up to three weeks in the refrigerator. Put the fennel into a plastic bag, which will help to keep it fresh and crisp.

Makes one glass

3 tomatoes

½ cucumber

1 stalk celery

1 fennel

1 green apple

Rinse the ingredients. Chop all the ingredients into small pieces and feed through a juicer. Pour into a glass and serve.

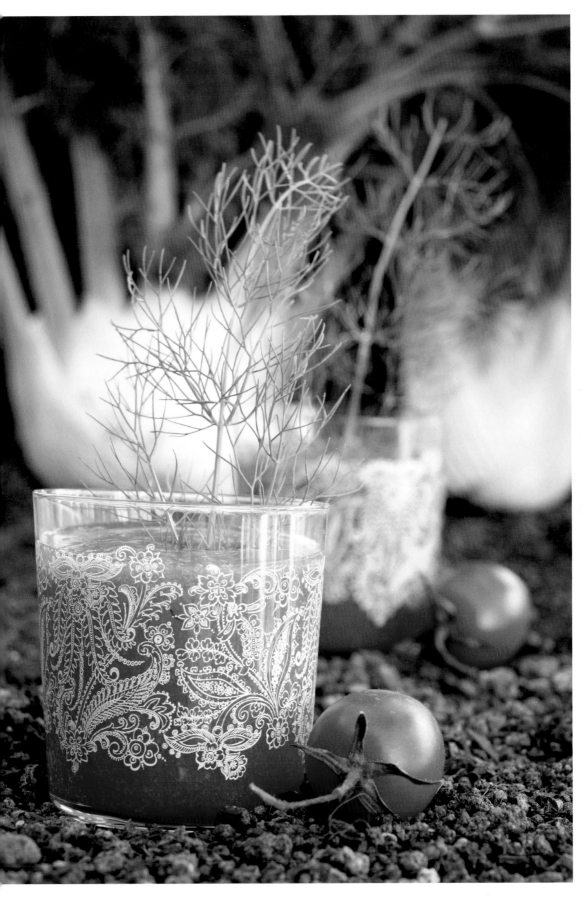

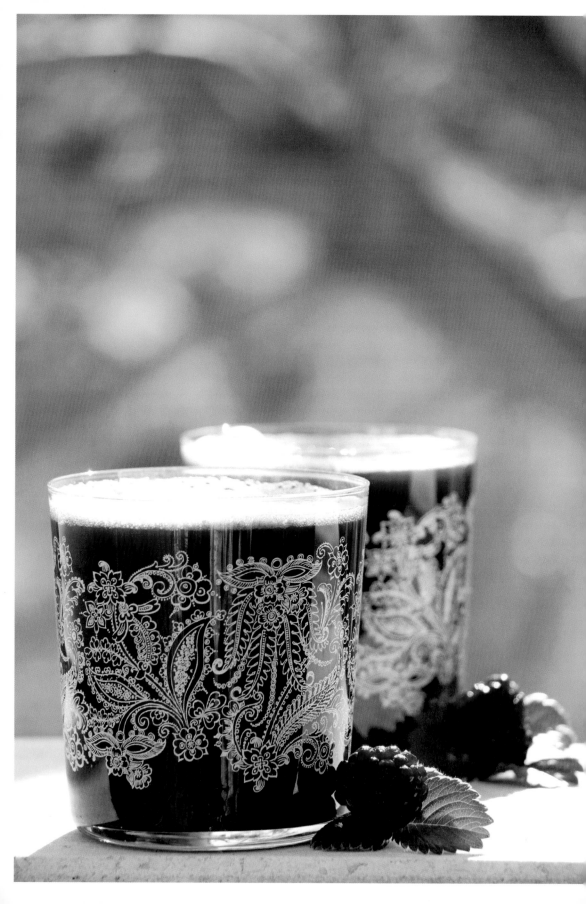

ANTIOXIDANT BOMB

Blackcurrants contain plenty of fiber, antioxidants, vitamins A, C, and K as well as folic acid. The seeds also contain gamma-linolenic acid, vitamin E, and essential polyunsaturated fatty acids, which, among other things, have been proven to lower blood cholesterol. For optimum health benefits, crush the seeds or take them in berry powder form.

The blackcurrant season in Europe and the US is in the months of June to August, so make sure to stock up and freeze.

Makes one glass

1 red beet

1 carrot

1 cup / 100 g blackcurrants, fresh or defrosted

1 cup / 100 g blueberries, fresh or defrosted

1 cup / 100 g blackberries, fresh or defrosted

1 handful basil

Rinse the beet and carrot, trim the tops and bottoms, chop into small pieces, and feed through a juicer. Transfer the juice into a blender and blend with the remaining ingredients for a smooth texture. Pour into a glass and serve.

DANDELION AND MELON JUICE

The milky sap of the dandelion contains many bitter-tasting compounds that stimulate the appetite, promote salivary production, and increase glandular secretion in the digestive tract and liver. In late summer, the root contains the highest level of these bitter-tasting compounds, whereas in the spring, the highest levels are found in the leaves. In addition to bitter-tasting compounds, the leaves contain vitamins B and C and potassium. Dandelion has a strong diuretic effect. In Germany and Austria, dandelion is prescribed for gallbladder complaints and liver diseases as well as for gout and rheumatism.

Dandelion is used for making dandelion wine or syrup. It also makes a delicious salad or a cup of tea. During the war years of the 1940s, the root was roasted and used as a coffee substitute. A 14-day diet consisting of fresh dandelion stalks is said to cure fatigue and weakness. The plant is also believed to cleanse the blood and fortify the body.

Makes one glass

1 bunch dandelion leaves

1 stalk celery

4 leaves kale

½ head broccoli

½ honeydew melon

Rinse all the ingredients. You do not have to peel the melon if it has a soft skin. Leave the nutritious seeds in. Chop all the ingredients into small pieces and feed through a juicer. Pour into a glass and serve.

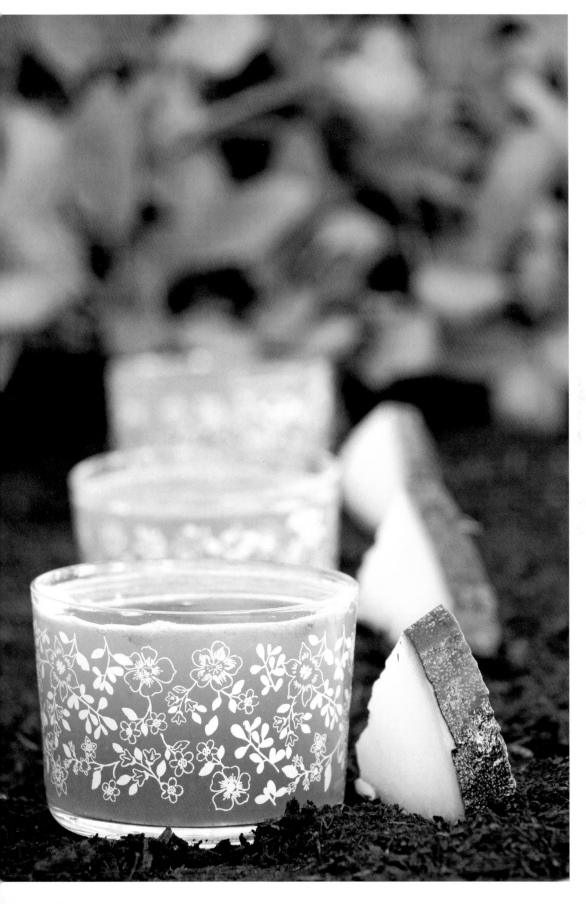

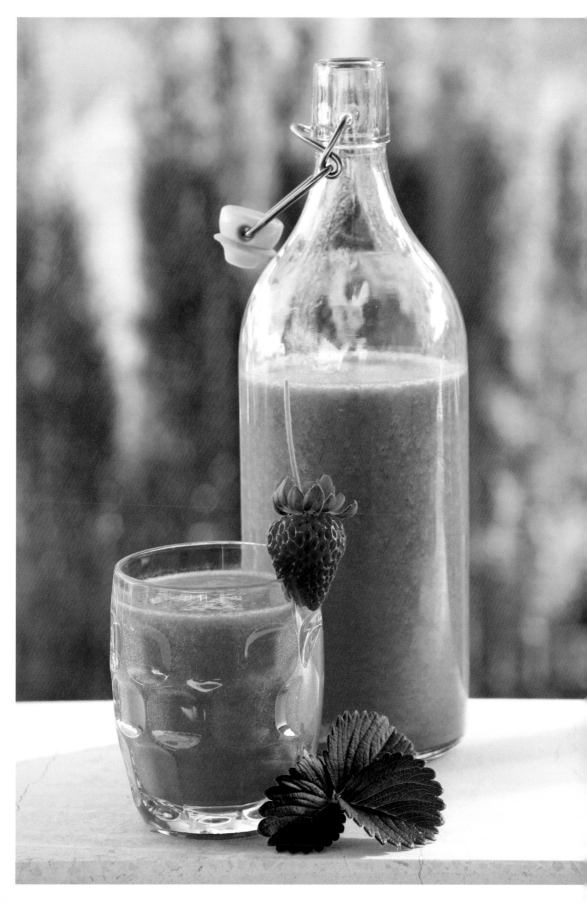

STRAWBERRY AND KOMBUCHA SMOOTHIE

Kombucha tea is a Chinese health drink with an ancient history. The tea was drunk as early as 200 BC and has, according to its proponents, many health-promoting properties, some of which are said to improve digestion and complexion and reduce body and joint pain. Kombucha also alleviates hunger and stomach and intestinal problems, such as gas, constipation, and the side effects of drug treatment. The drink is also said to boost immunity, preventing colds and flu. Among other beneficial ingredients, kombucha tea contains lactic bacteria, acetic acid, polysaccharide, and vitamins C, E, K, B1, B2, B3, B6, and B12 as well as the following minerals: iron, sodium, manganese, magnesium, potassium, copper, and zinc.

Kombucha tea is made from the fermented kombucha fungus (also called the Volga or tea fungus). The fungus varies in color, ranging from light and transparent to tea-brown. The drink is prepared by combining a yeast and bacterial culture with sugar and tea (black, green, or oolong) and allowing it to ferment for around 10 days. Kombucha tea is available in health food stores and comes in a variety of flavors. If you can get hold of a kombucha culture, you can also produce and flavor your own tea.

According to traditional Chinese medicine, kombucha tea is considered an immortality drink and the elixir of life.

Makes one glass

½ lemon

2 cups / 200 g strawberries, frozen

1⅓ cups / 200 g watermelon

generous ¾ cup / 200 ml kombucha tea

1 tbsp agave syrup

Squeeze the juice from the lemon. Peel the watermelon if the rind is thick, leaving the seeds in. Chop into small pieces. Blend everything till you get a smooth mixture. Pour into a glass and serve.

THE CITRUS KICK

Most people probably know that the orange is high in vitamin C, but what is perhaps less well known is that it also contains other beneficial substances that are not provided by an effervescent tablet. In addition to strengthening immunity, decreasing blood pressure, and preventing colds and infections, the orange offers extra protection against eye disease, rheumatism, cardiovascular diseases, and cancer. Also, the vitamin C contained in an orange is important for revitalizing the skin.

Vitamin C helps the body to absorb more nutrients, such as iron, zinc, copper, calcium, and vitamin B9 (folic acid). Vitamin C also has an antioxidant effect on other substances in the body and helps to break down harmful free radicals. Vitamin C cannot be stored in the body and must therefore be supplied every day.

Makes one glass

1 grapefruit, pink or red

1 orange

1 lemon

1 pear

Rinse all the ingredients. Remove the zest of the citrus fruits, taking care not to remove the nutritious white pith beneath. Chop into small pieces and feed through a juicer. Pour into a glass and serve.

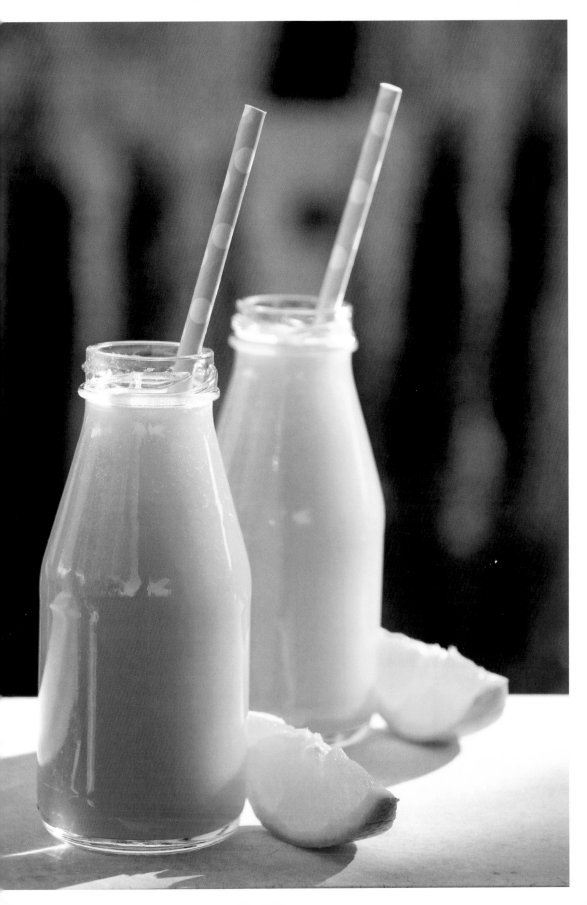

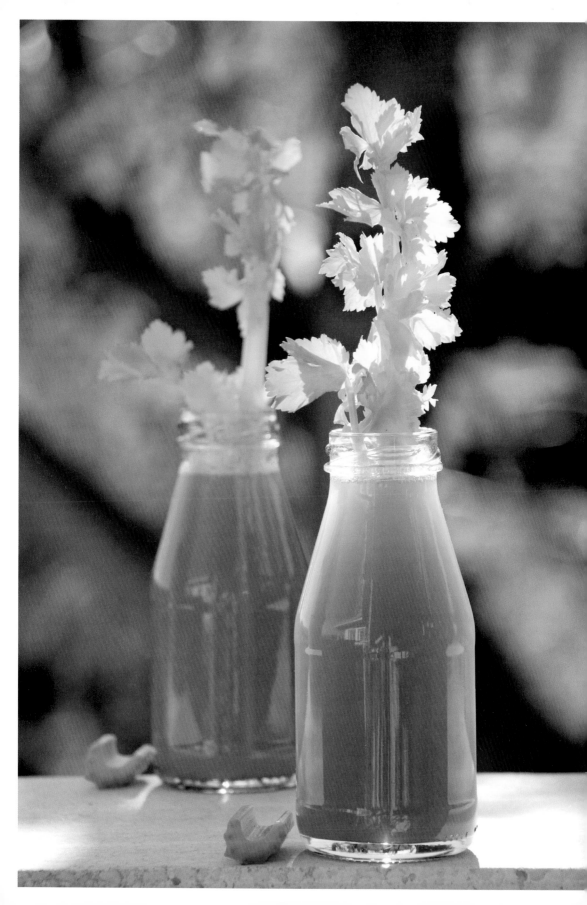

MELON AND CELERY JUICE

Celery is high in potassium and is an excellent source of vitamin C, vitamin A, calcium, and protein. Celery is believed to be helpful in counteracting high blood pressure. The bulk of the vitamin C, calcium, and potassium is contained in the green leaves, which should be used within a couple of days, as otherwise they will wither and the vitamins will be lost.

When shopping for celery, look out for straight, rigid stalks that snap when bent and for leaves that have not started to turn yellow or wilt. Store celery in the refrigerator in a sealed container or wrapped in a plastic bag or damp cloth. Celery should not be stored at room temperature for too long, as it wilts quickly because of its high water content. If it starts to droop, splash some water on the celery and put it back in the refrigerator, where it will regain its crispness.

This recipe is high in protein and is ideal for recovery after a hard workout.

Makes one glass

1 lime

2 stalks celery

½ Galia melon

¼ head Savoy cabbage

Rinse all the ingredients. Remove the zest of the lime, taking care not to remove the nutritious white pith beneath. Chop the ingredients into small pieces and feed through a juicer. Pour into a glass and serve.

SPROUT SMOOTHIE

A sprout marks the beginning of life and contains valuable substances, such as vegetable protein, unsaturated fatty acids, and essential minerals. When a seed sprouts, the content of vital B and E vitamins increases enormously. These substances are most needed after the winter in order to increase resilience and fend off spring fatigue. Sprouts are a great and delicious addition to a smoothie, juice, or tasty salad; they are wholesome eaten on a crispbread sandwich or used in Asian cooking, and they are not difficult to grow. There are many different varieties of sprouts, the principle being that any seed can be sprouted (e.g. alfalfa, fenugreek, mung beans, wheat, broccoli, and radish. Buckwheat, millet, quinoa, sunflower, linseed, and chia seeds are also easy to sprout).

Sprouting seeds are available in health food stores. The growing instructions are usually given on the back of the seed packet, the method varying depending on the type of seed you wish to sprout. There are also special sprouting jars/trays, where you can grow several different sprout varieties at the same time. Sprouts will keep for 2–3 days in the fridge.

Makes one glass

generous ¾ cup / 85 g fresh, mild-tasting sprouts

½ cucumber

1 green apple

1 pear

Rinse all the ingredients (apart from the sprouts, if growing them at home). Chop into small pieces. Feed the cucumber, apple, and pear through a juicer. Transfer the juice to a blender, add the sprouts, and blend thoroughly. Pour into a glass and serve.

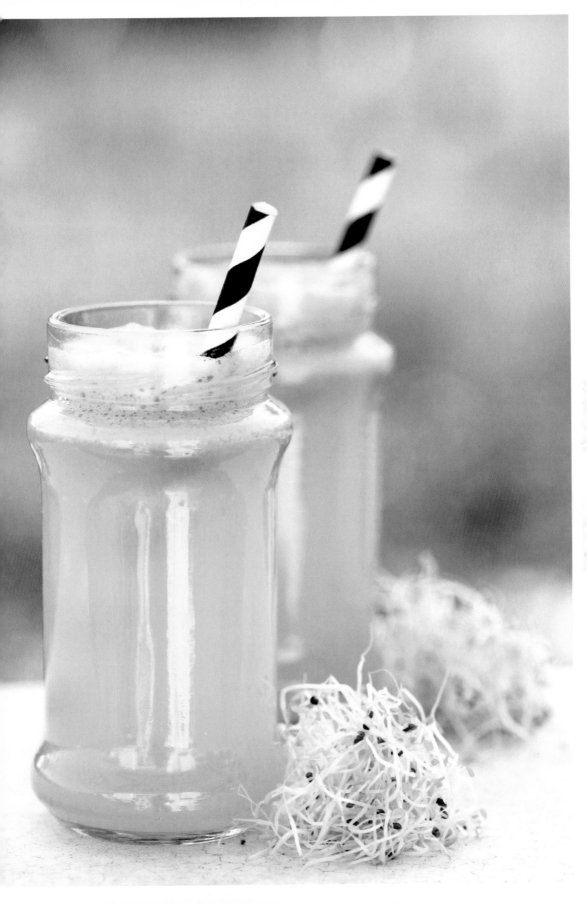

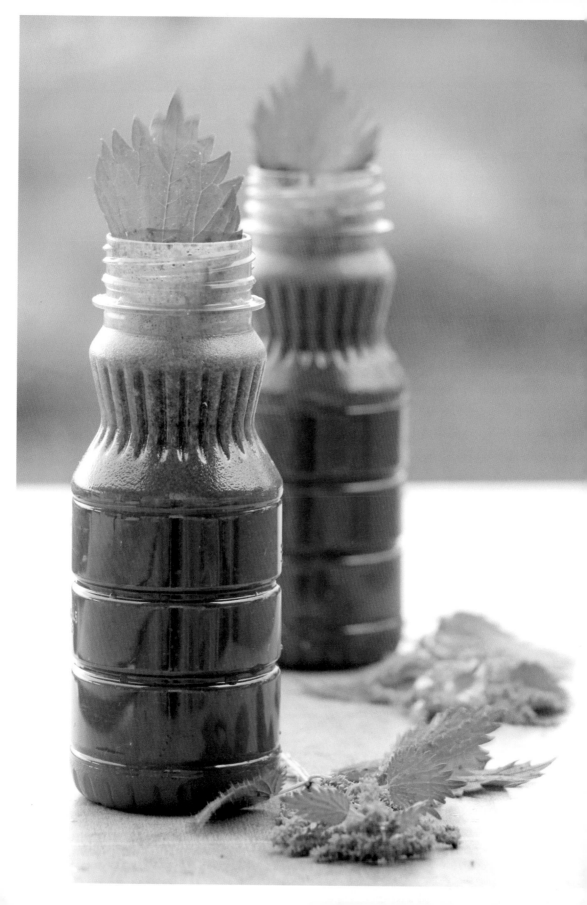

STINGING NETTLE AND PINEAPPLE JUICE

Most people know about the stinging nettle. Is there anyone that has not been stung by it?

Few plants are as beneficial as the nettle. In the 16th and 17th centuries, it was used as medicine against paralysis, rheumatism, scurvy, tuberculosis, cough, and baldness (the leaves being hairy!). Unfortunately, the treatments did not frequently produce the desired result, even though the vitamins and minerals contained in the nettle were certainly much needed to supplement people's diets. Nowadays, however, the nettle is believed to purify the blood and to have a bracing effect.

The first leaves of spring contain the highest amount of nutrients. The nettle is primarily rich in chlorophyll, but also in beta-carotene, calcium, potassium, magnesium, iron, silicon, manganese, flavonoids, provitamin A, and vitamins C, K, and B, as well as folic acid. Nettle powder is easy to use and is available in health food stores.

Makes one glass

1 lime

½ pineapple

1 handful nettles or 1 tbsp nettle powder

1 apple

Rinse the ingredients. Remove the zest of the lime, taking care not to remove the nutritious white pith beneath. Remove the leafy crown of the pineapple and cut away the hard skin. Chop all the ingredients into small pieces and feed through a juicer. Pour into a glass and serve.

CARROT, SWEET POTATO, AND PARSLEY JUICE

The fresh leaves of parsley contain iron, calcium, and magnesium, among other nutrients, as well as vitamins A and C. Just ⅕ ounce / 5 g parsley meets our daily vitamin A requirement and 1 ounce / 30 g our daily requirement of vitamin C. Parsley is a diuretic, antispasmodic, and hypotensive, and it reduces the risk of cardiac arrhythmia (atrial fibrillation). Parsley also stimulates the appetite and raises the metabolic rate. Chewing parsley freshens up breath (it helps against garlic odor, for example).

Sweet potatoes are packed with antioxidants and are rich in vitamins C and E and beta-carotene, as well as in the minerals iron, copper, folate, and potassium.

Makes one glass

1 lime

1 apple

1 stalk celery

2 carrots

1 sweet potato

1 generous handful parsley

Rinse all the ingredients. Remove the zest of the lime, taking care not to remove the nutritious white pith beneath. Trim the tops and bottoms of the root vegetables. Chop all the ingredients into small pieces and feed through a juicer. Pour into a glass and serve.

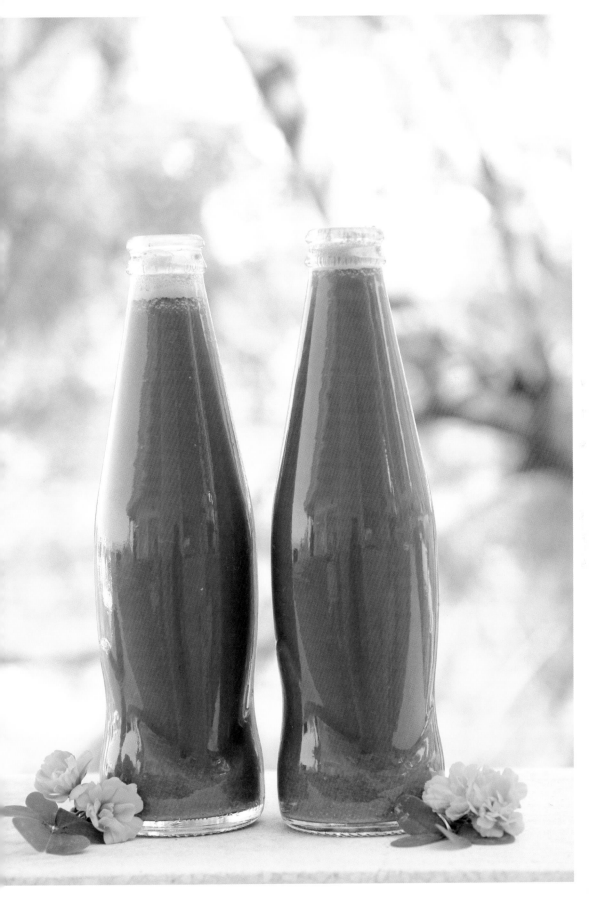

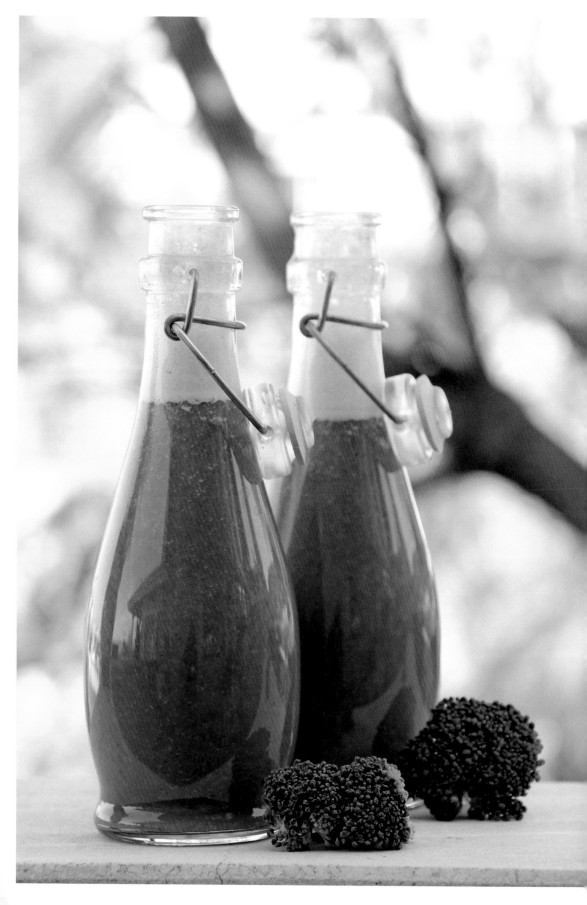

BROCCOLI AND PEAR JUICE

For vegans and other people who do not eat dairy, broccoli is a valuable source of calcium. Calcium fortifies bones and is important for the muscles to function normally. Broccoli contains plenty of folic acid and vitamins A, C, and K as well as fiber. It also contains a certain amount of vitamins B6, B1, B2, B3, and E as well as iron, potassium, magnesium, and zinc.

Makes one glass

1 lime

1 handful sunflower sprouts (or other sprouts)

1 handful spinach

½ head broccoli

2 pears

Rinse all the ingredients. Remove the zest of the lime, taking care not to remove the nutritious white pith beneath. Chop all the ingredients into small pieces and feed through a juicer. Pour into a glass and serve.

PEAR AND MINT JUICE

Pears contain twice as much fiber as apples but have a shorter shelf life, so it's best to buy unripe pears and store them in the refrigerator for a few days before use. If you want to speed up the ripening process, they can be stored in a paper bag with an apple—apples produce ethylene gas, which makes other fruit ripen faster.

Fiber is essential in our diet—it helps to keep blood sugar levels down and aids digestion. A fiber-rich diet reduces the risk of cancer and also combats high cholesterol. In addition to fiber, pears are rich in potassium, riboflavin, and vitamins A and C.

Makes one glass

1 lime

5 stalks celery

½ cucumber

2 pears

1 handful mint

Rinse the ingredients. Remove the zest of the lime, taking care not to remove the nutritious white pith beneath. When feeding the ingredients through a juicer, make sure you alternate the mint (both twigs and leaves) with the other ingredients, as that will ensure you get more juice from it. Pour into a glass and serve.

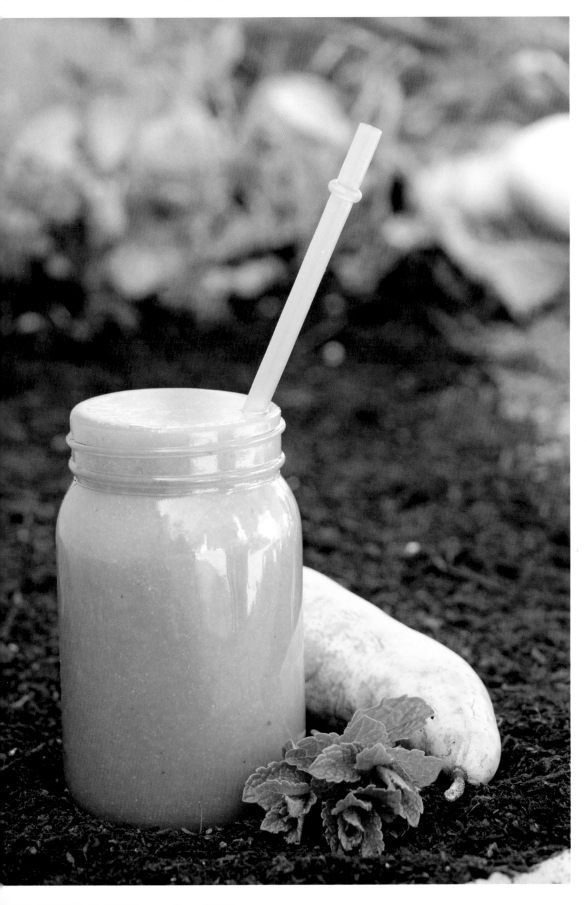

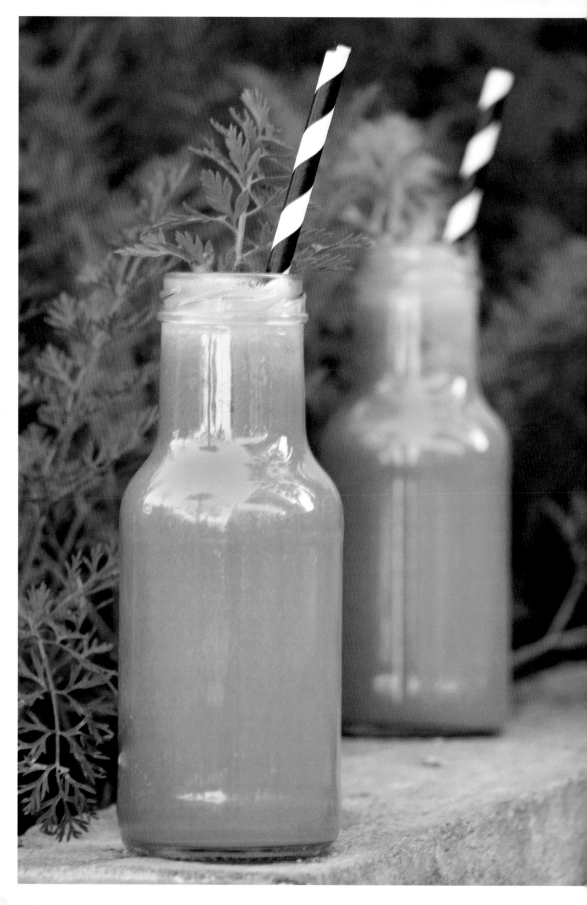

SPICY CARROT JUICE

Chili pepper may seem addictive. This is because capsaicin, the substance that makes chili pepper hot, increases the production of endorphins in the body. Endorphins have an analgesic effect and produce feelings of wellbeing and relaxation, so it's no wonder that people sometimes crave chili pepper.

Cayenne pepper is a type of chili pepper that has been shown to have several beneficial properties:

» It raises the metabolic rate, is an expectorant, and is generally good for digestion.

» It cleanses the body of toxins and is both bactericidal and analgesic.

» It lowers blood pressure and is useful in the fight against cardiovascular disease and cancer.

» It thins the blood and is beneficial for angina sufferers (and, just like garlic, it dilates the arteries).

» It can even be sprinkled onto a wound to stop bleeding.

Makes one glass

4 carrots

1 oz / 25 g fresh ginger

¾ oz / 20 g fresh turmeric or
1 tsp turmeric powder
(optional)

½ cucumber

1 apple

1 pinch cayenne pepper

Rinse the ingredients. Chop them into small pieces and feed through a juicer. Sprinkle the cayenne pepper on top. Pour into a glass and serve.

RED BEET DETOX JUICE

Surely you're not throwing away the best part of the red beet? The greens are the most nutritious part, so be sure to use them. If you have bought organically grown beets or grow them yourself, you can safely use the greens in this detox juice. Ask for extra greens if you're buying direct from a grower.

Beet greens are very similar to chard, in terms of both flavor and appearance.

Makes one glass

1 lemon

2 red beets

2 stalks celery

⅓ cucumber

⅓ oz / 10 g ginger

1 handful parsley

Rinse the ingredients. Remove the zest of the lemon, taking care not to remove the nutritious white pith beneath. Trim the tops and bottoms of the beets. Chop all the ingredients into small pieces. When feeding the ingredients through a juicer, make sure you alternate the parsley (both twigs and leaves) with the other ingredients, as that will ensure you get more juice from it. Pour into a glass and serve.

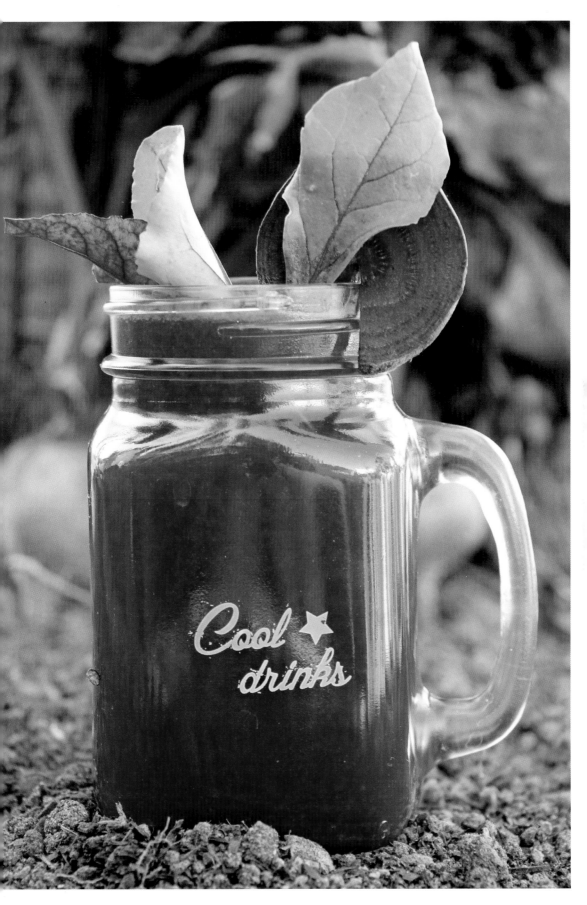

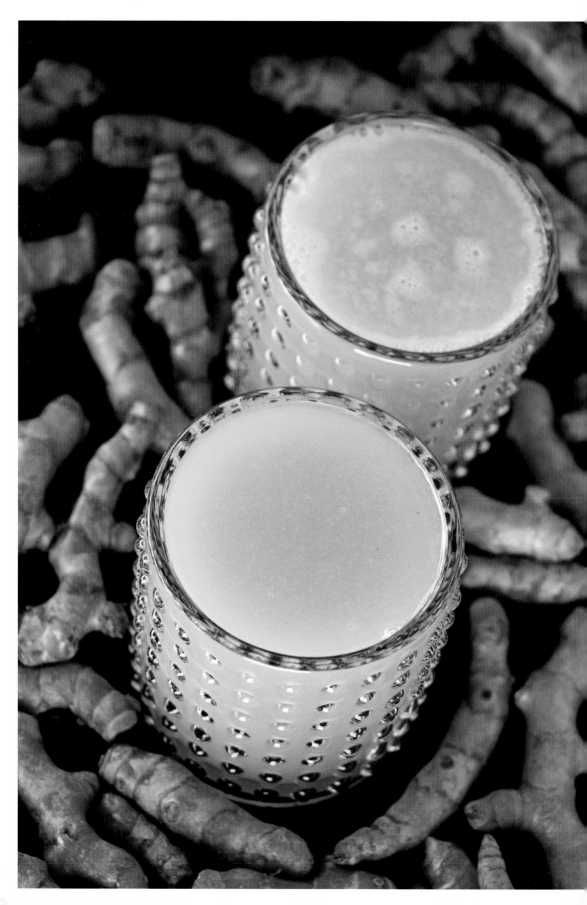

MANGO AND TURMERIC JUICE

Mango is the national fruit of India and Pakistan. It is rich in several groups of antioxidants, such as beta-carotene, vitamin C, and potassium. Beta-carotene is converted to vitamin A in the body, which is good for eyesight, bones, skin, mucous membranes, and immunity. Vitamin C strengthens blood vessels, skin, teeth, and bones.

Like cashew nuts, mango (the skin, in particular) contains urushiol. Allergy sufferers should take some care—at least when peeling the skin.

In season, you can freeze mangoes in single serving packets. It is much cheaper and tastier to eat frozen fruit than fruit that has been picked unripe, stored for a long time, and sprayed with various agents to stay fresh for months. Freshly harvested fruit is always best, but freshly harvested fruit that is frozen direct is also good for you. Smell and gently squeeze a mango to see if it is ripe.

Makes one glass

1 lime
1 grapefruit
1 mango
½ oz / 15 g fresh turmeric or
1 tsp turmeric powder

Rinse the ingredients. Remove the zest of the lime and grapefruit, taking care not to remove the nutritious white pith beneath. Peel the mango and remove the pit. Use gloves or peel the fresh turmeric holding it inside a plastic bag, otherwise you won't be able to remove the yellow color from your hands for a few days. Feed all the ingredients into a juicer. Pour into a glass and serve.

Or make a smoothie. To do so, squeeze the juice of the lime using a citrus juicer. Whizz everything in a blender and serve.

SPINACH AND APPLE SMOOTHIE

Spinach is a fantastic vegetable and one rich in antioxidants. The leaves are incredibly nutritious and, among other nutrients, contain vitamins A, C, E, K, and vitamin B9 (folic acid). Spinach is also rich in copper, iron, magnesium, calcium, chlorophyll, fiber, and other beneficial substances.

Spinach has a high inorganic nitrate content, which is believed to improve physical performance and muscle growth. Studies have shown that spinach makes the mitochondria—the energy hubs of the muscle cells—more efficient, thereby reducing the body's need for oxygen during physical exertion. Spinach is also believed to fight cancer and reduce high blood pressure. It can also help to alleviate the symptoms of gastric ulcers.

Makes one glass

1 lime

2 handfuls spinach

3 apples

½ avocado

Rinse all the ingredients. Remove the zest of the lime, taking care not to remove the nutritious white pith beneath. Chop the apples into small pieces. Feed the lime, spinach, and apples through a juicer and transfer the juice into a blender. Scoop out the flesh of the avocado straight into the blender and blend everything to a creamy consistency. Pour into a glass and serve.

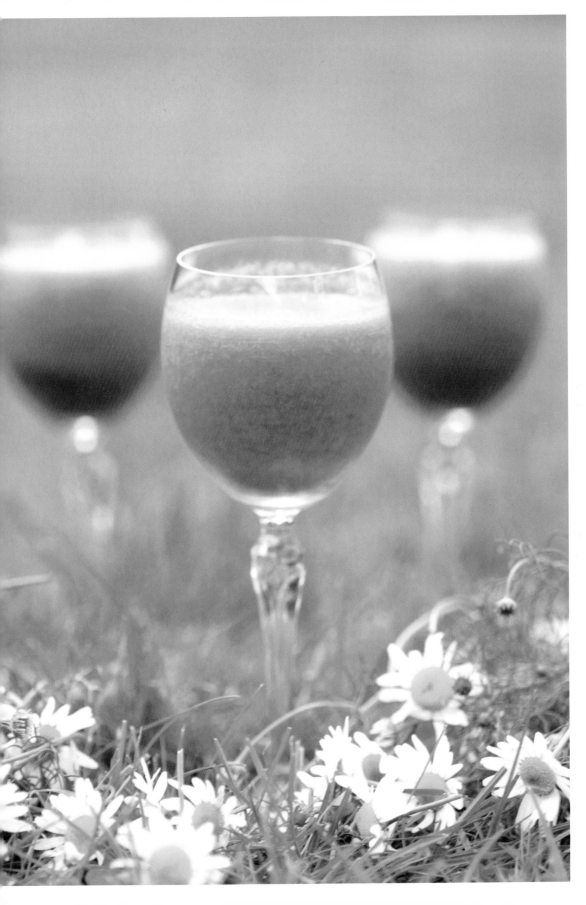

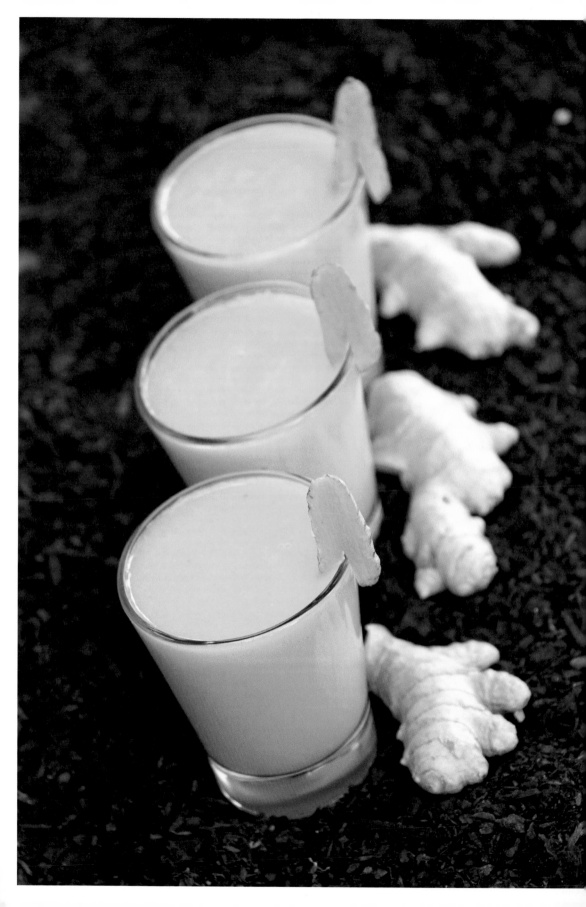

TURMERIC AND GINGER SHOT

Fresh turmeric can be grown in the same way as ginger. In early spring, plant the root in a flowerpot, leave it outdoors during the summer, and harvest in the fall. If you are struggling to peel the root, you can freeze it and peel it frozen. If you wash and scrub the skin properly, you do not need to peel it. Take care when using fresh turmeric, as it tends to leave stubborn smudges on both your hands and kitchen surfaces and is very hard to remove. Use gloves or peel it holding it inside a plastic bag.

Makes one shot

1 tsp agave syrup

1 lemon

1 apple

¾ oz / 20 g fresh ginger

¾ oz / 20 g fresh turmeric or 1 tsp turmeric powder

Pour the agave syrup into a glass. Remove the zest of the lemon, taking care not to remove the nutritious white pith beneath. Feed the apple, lemon, ginger, and turmeric through a juicer. Pour the juice into the glass with the agave syrup, stir, and serve. Cheers!

SPIRULINA SHOT

Spirulina is 60–70 percent protein, which makes it six times more protein-rich than eggs and three times more so than steak. Its protein consists of 18 different amino acids, 8 of which are essential for human health. Spirulina also contains many essential minerals, including calcium, magnesium, sodium, potassium, phosphorus, iodine, selenium, iron, copper, and zinc; and a broad spectrum of B vitamins, e.g. B1, B2, B5, B6, B11, and B12, as well as vitamins C and E. Its content of beta-carotene, which is converted into vitamin A in the body, is 15 times higher than that of carrots and 40–60 times higher than that of spinach.

Makes one shot

1 orange

1 tsp spirulina powder

Rinse the orange and squeeze out the juice. Pour into a glass and mix in the spirulina powder. Drink at once! Perhaps not the most delicious drink you have ever tasted, but it's oh, so good for you!

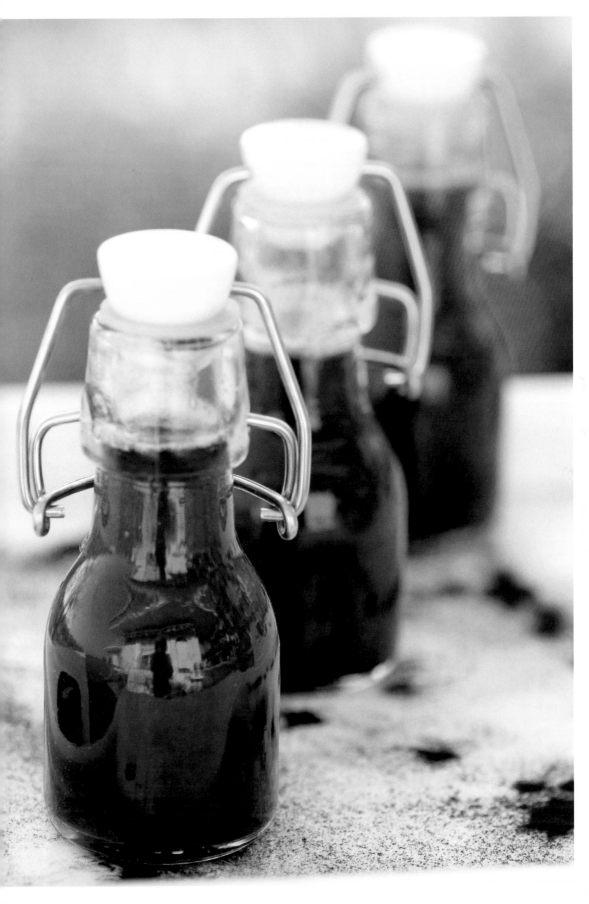

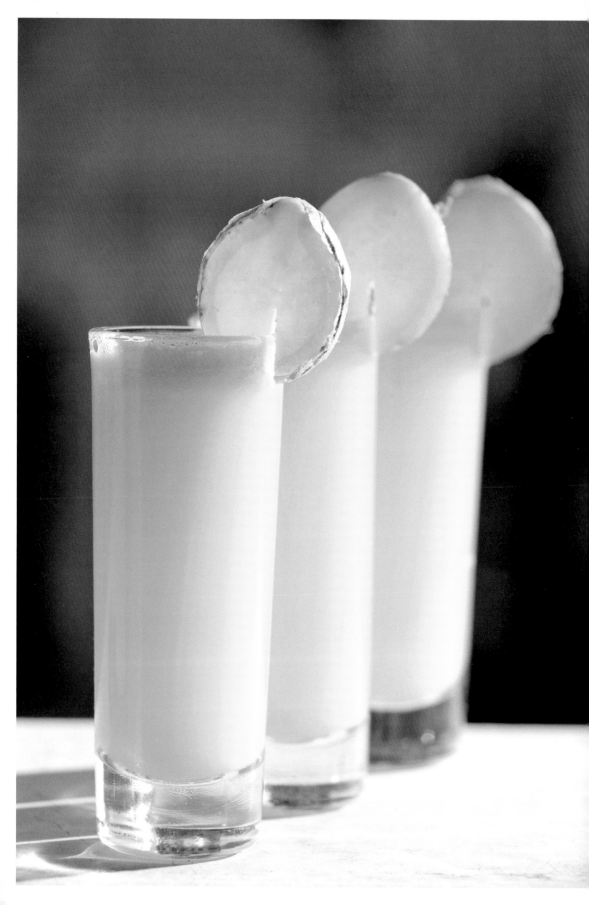

APPLE AND GINGER SHOT

Ginger strengthens immunity and is an anti-inflammatory. It has a positive effect on rheumatoid arthritis, strengthens the heart, stimulates breathing, and improves blood circulation. Ginger relieves nausea and is also effective against motion sickness.

Makes one shot

1 lime

1 apple

ginger—as much as you can handle

Rinse all the ingredients. Remove the zest of the lime, taking care not to remove the nutritious white pith beneath. Chop the apple into small pieces. Feed all the ingredients through a juicer. Pour into a glass and serve.

RED BEET AND GARLIC SHOT

Garlic contains, among other ingredients, alliin, allicin, silicic acid, and vitamins A, B, and C as well as small amounts of sodium, selenium, iodine, potassium, iron, calcium, phosphorus, zinc, chromium, magnesium, and copper. It lowers blood pressure and blood sugar and reduces cholesterol and triglycerides in the blood. Garlic also contains anti-inflammatory, antibiotic, and antifungal properties. It is both an antispasmodic and an expectorant and inhibits bacterial fermentation in the gut. It is also said to relieve menopausal symptoms.

There are a lot of tricks to get rid of garlic odor on your breath. One of the most common ones is to chew parsley, basil, mint, or thyme.

Makes one shot

1 red beet

garlic—as much as you can handle

Himalayan salt (optional)

Rinse the beet, trim the top and the bottom, and chop it into small pieces. Alternate the garlic and beet as you feed them through a juicer. Pour the juice into a shot glass and add a pinch of Himalayan salt if desired.

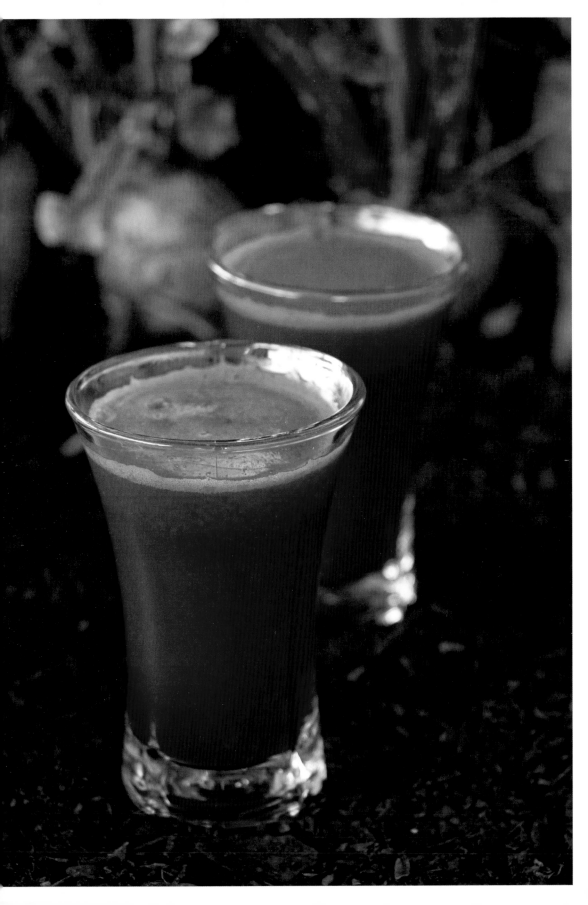

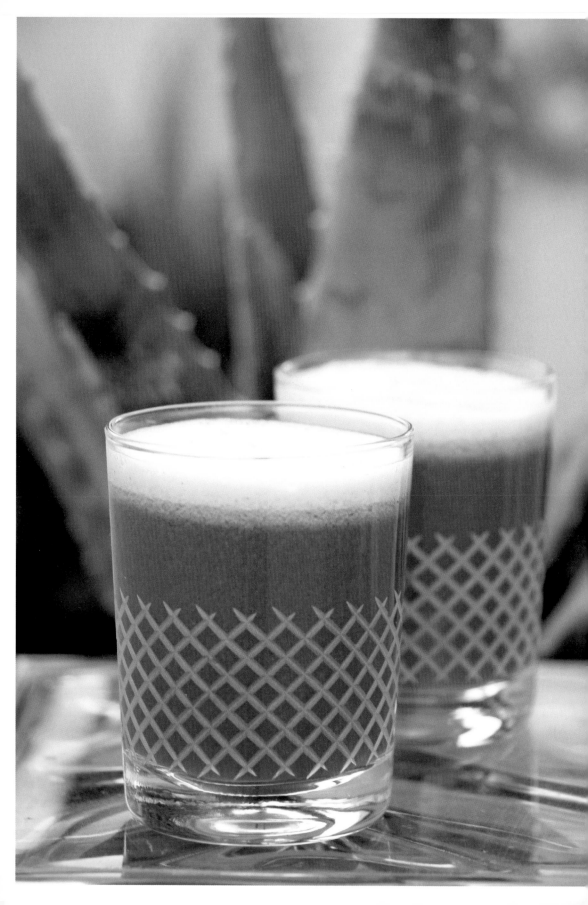

ALOE VERA AND APPLE SHOT

Aloe barbadensis is thought to be one of the oldest medicinal plants known to humankind. It has been used for thousands of years in folk medicine around the world. Nowadays, aloe vera is added to many different drinks and concentrated juices, but never in any significant quantity. Make sure, therefore, that you read the ingredients list so you know how much aloe vera there is in the product you are consuming. Aloe vera juice should contain a pure, concentrated, and cold-pressed juice from cultivated *Aloe barbadensis* plants.

Aloe vera is known by a variety of names including Venus's gift, medicinal plant, doctor in the pot, miracle plant, magic wand from the heavens, and plant for burns.

In large quantities, fresh aloe vera can have a laxative effect, so do not consume too much.

Makes one shot

1 green apple

2 tsp aloe vera juice

Rinse the apple, chop it into small pieces, and feed through a juicer. Pour the apple juice into a glass and stir in the aloe vera juice.

SHOT FOR COLDS

Our immune system is one of the body's most advanced mechanisms, but most of us do not pay any attention to it until we get ill. The immune system's job is to protect us from the onslaught of viruses, bacteria, and microorganisms.

Most people get a cold during the winter. Colds are caused by viruses and, since we are surrounded by approximately 200 cold viruses at any given time, it is important that your immunity is strong and that it can protect you, not just from the common cold, but also from severe infections and diseases.

By eating healthily and leading a healthy lifestyle, you can strengthen your immunity on a regular basis by means of relatively simple solutions.

Makes one shot

1 tsp honey

1 small chili pepper (or a pinch chili powder)

½ lemon

½ orange

1 clove garlic

⅓ oz / 10 g fresh ginger

⅓ oz / 10 g fresh turmeric or ½ tsp turmeric powder

Rinse those ingredients that need rinsing. I prefer to leave the skin of the ginger and turmeric on. Place the honey and chili powder (if using) into a glass. Remove the zest of the orange and lemon, taking care not to remove the nutritious white pith beneath. Feed all the ingredients, apart from the honey and chili powder, through a juicer. Pour the juice into a glass and stir.

Make triple the quantity if you have a really bad cold. Store the remaining two portions in a glass bottle in the refrigerator and drink a shot every three hours.

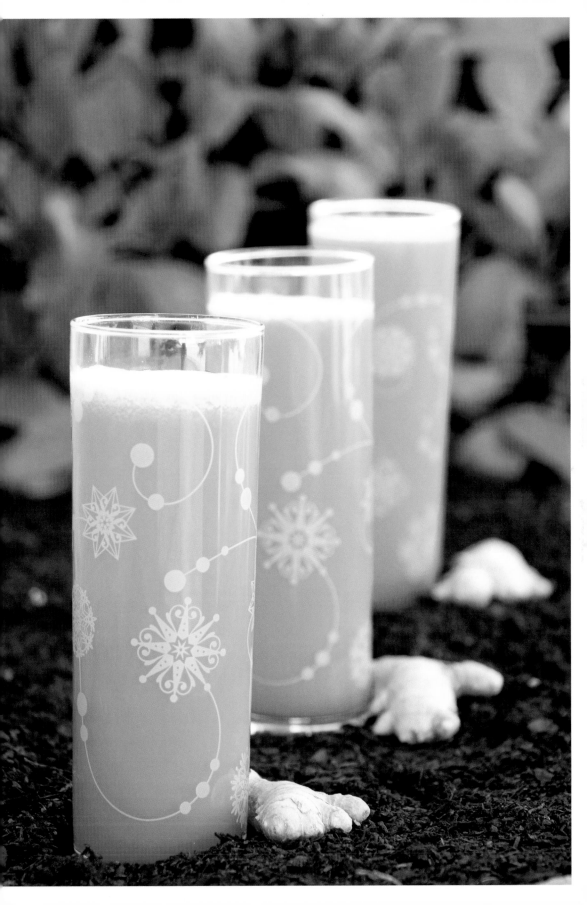

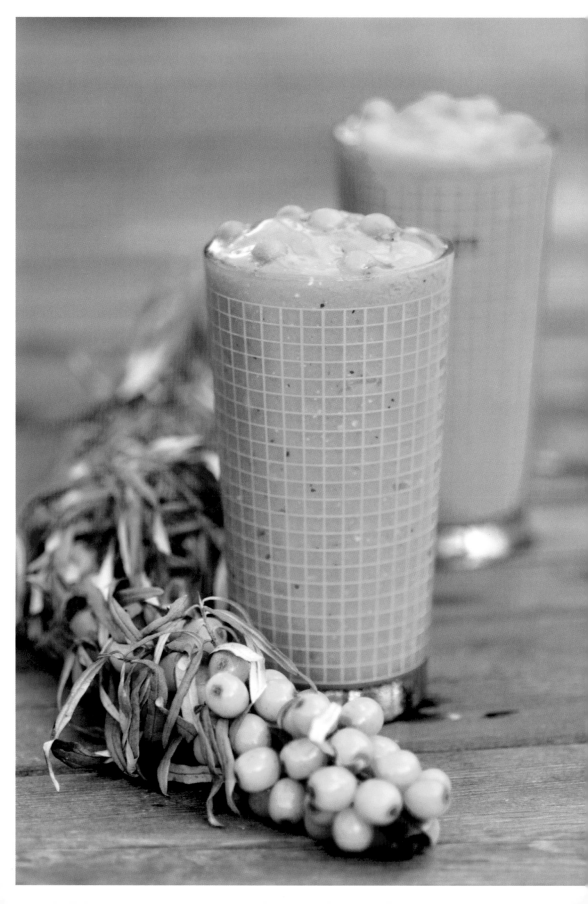

SEA BUCKTHORN AND ORANGE SHOT

It is said that a single small sea buckthorn berry contains as much vitamin C as a whole orange. However, the vitamin C in sea buckthorn varies depending on variety and ripeness. Sea buckthorn contains vitamin B12, which is rarely found in plants and is, therefore, particularly important for vegetarians, but it also contains vitamins B1, B2, B3 (niacin), B6, and B9 (folic acid), as well as pantothenic acid, biotin, and vitamins E and K.

Makes one shot

1 orange

1 cup / 200 g frozen sea buckthorn or 2 tsp sea buckthorn powder

a few ice cubes

Rinse the orange and remove the zest, taking care not to remove the nutritious white pith beneath. Blend all the ingredients to make a frosty smoothie shot. Pour into glasses and serve.

COCONUT AND MAQUI BERRY SHOT

Maqui berries are native to Patagonia, southern Chile. The berries rank high on the ORAC (Oxygen Radical Absorbance Capacity) list, which compares the antioxidant effect of different foods. Maqui berries provide four times the antioxidant protection provided by blueberries and double that of acai berries. Antioxidants strengthen immunity, are anti-inflammatory, and balance blood sugar. In addition, the berries are effective against free radicals, protecting the cells of the body from oxidative stress and fighting premature aging. Maqui berries are also bursting with flavonoids, polyphenols, and vitamins A, C, and E, as well as calcium, iron, and potassium.

Makes one shot

1 tsp coconut oil

1 tsp blueberry powder

1 tsp maqui berry powder

3½ tbsp / 50 ml coconut milk

Combine all the ingredients in a blender and blend till smooth. Pour into a glass and serve. Healthy and super-scrumptious!

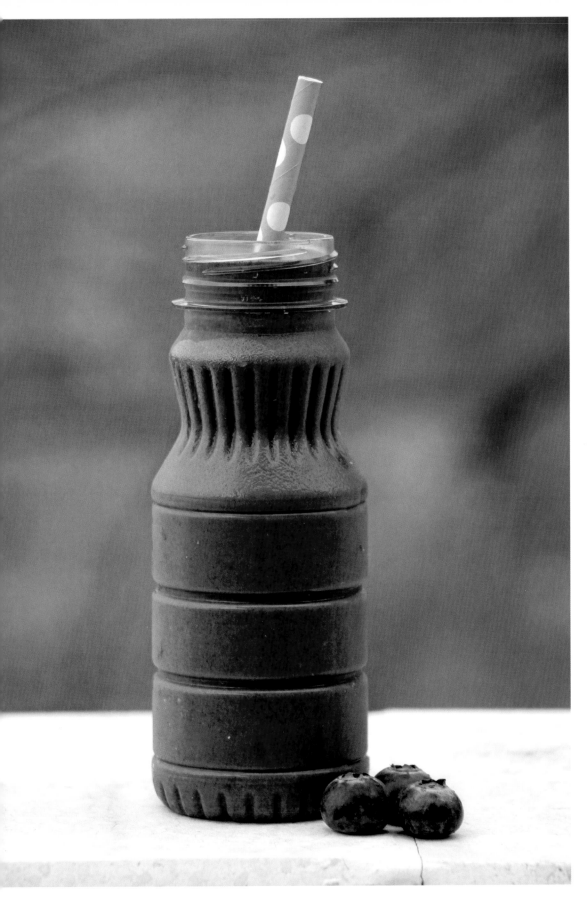

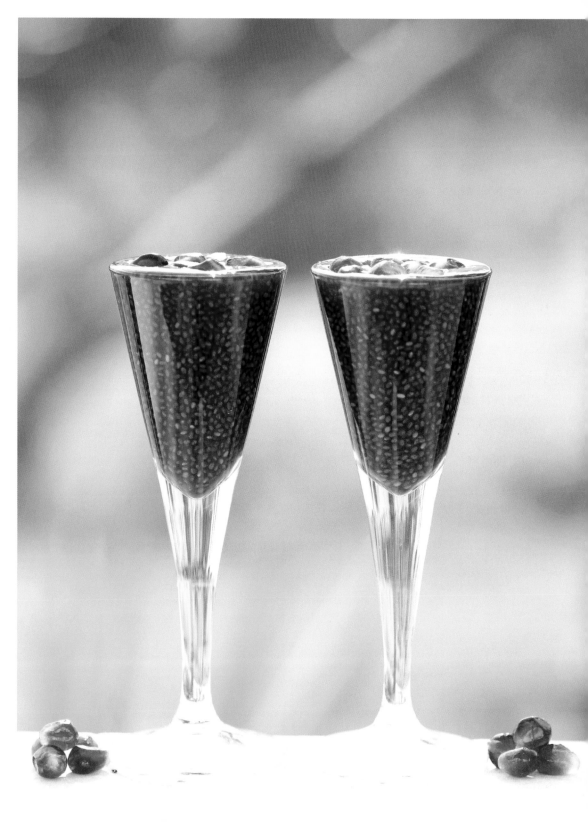

CHIA SHOT

Chia seeds are a true superfood. A portion of 3½ ounces / 100 g contains 1 ounce / 31 g fat, as much as ¾ ounce / 20 g of which is made up of linolenic acid. Two teaspoons of chia seeds contain more omega-3 fatty acids than a standard-size salmon fillet. Omega-3 fatty acids are important for the body's hormonal balance and may have an anti-inflammatory effect. In addition, the seeds are rich in minerals, such as magnesium, potassium, and zinc.

A portion of 3½ ounces / 100 g of chia seeds also contains ¾ ounce / 21 g protein, which contains up to 18 amino acids. In other words, it is an important source of vegetable protein.

Lastly, chia seeds also contain large amounts of water-soluble fiber, which improves gut function and helps to keep blood sugar in balance.

Makes one shot

1 pomegranate

1 tsp passion fruit powder (optional)

2 tsp chia seeds

water (optional)

Rinse the pomegranate, cut it in half and squeeze the juice using a simple citrus press. Pour the juice into a glass and add the passion fruit powder and chia seeds. Stir and leave to stand in the refrigerator (covered with plastic wrap) for 20–30 minutes. Chia seeds absorb liquid, turning them into a jelly, so if the shot is too thick, dilute it with a little water to make it go down more easily. Or eat it with a spoon.

POMEGRANATE AND RED BEET SHOT

Pomegranate is a superfruit and has been grown for thousands of years. It originates from Persia. Pomegranate is particularly rich in folic acid and antioxidants, e.g. vitamin C, carotene, gallocatechin, and anthocyanins (which give the pomegranate its characteristic pink color). Antioxidants strengthen the body's cells and help to fight disease. Folic acid is important for new cell growth and plays a key role in the formation of red blood cells.

Do you struggle to get those delicious seeds from a pomegranate? Here's a tip: roll the pomegranate back and forth on a hard surface and cut it in half. Then hold each half over a bowl, seeds facing down, and tap the skin with a wooden spoon—and there you have it!

Pomegranates are available fresh during fall and winter, but you can also use frozen or dried seeds when pomegranates are not in season.

Makes one shot

1 small red beet

1 pomegranate

Rinse the ingredients. Trim the top and bottom of the beet. Cut the pomegranate in half. Carefully peel away the skin and empty the seeds into a bowl. Process the beet and pomegranate seeds in a juicer. Pour into a glass and serve. This is a real dark-red energy bomb!

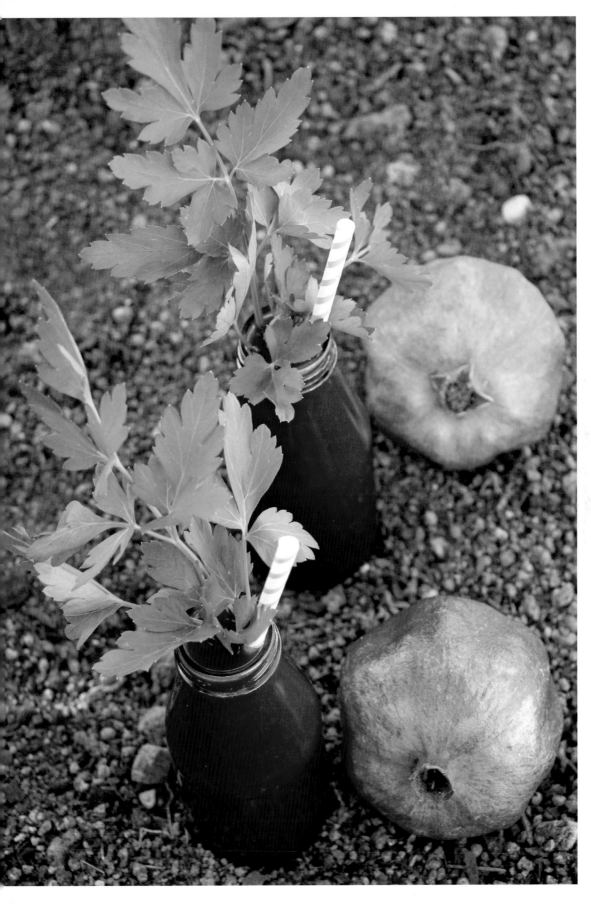

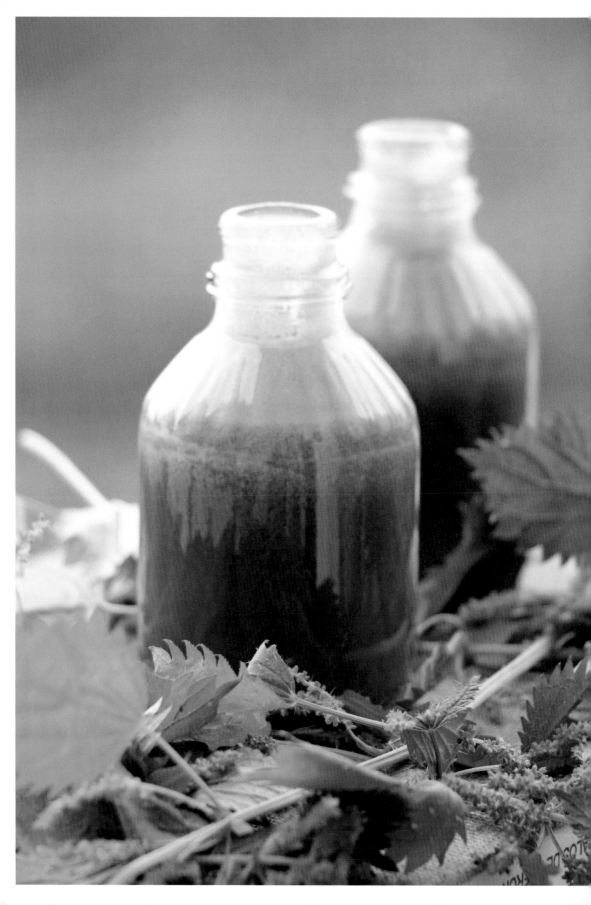

STINGING NETTLE AND PEAR SHOT

Chlorophyll, which is found in abundance in the stinging nettle, has a chemical structure similar to our own hemoglobin. This is why it helps to improve the transportation of oxygen and nutrients to body cells.

A teaspoon of nettle powder is said to meet your whole daily recommended amount of vitamin C.

Makes one shot

½ lime

1 large pear

1 tsp stinging nettle powder or a handful nettles

Rinse the fruit. Remove the zest of the lime, taking care not to remove the nutritious white pith beneath. Chop the pear into pieces. Feed the lime and pear through a juicer. Pour the juice into a glass and stir in the nettle powder.

This shot provides a green energy kick in the morning or in the middle of the day!

ROSEHIP AND ORANGE SHOT

In the past, rosehip was used in folk medicine to prevent scurvy, a condition caused by vitamin C deficiency. Rosehip is also considered to be effective against constipation, fatigue, joint problems, diverticulosis, emphysema, ear problems, hemorrhoids, urinary bladder problems, colic, and stiffness; as well as back, bone, feet, and neck problems. The use of rosehip in traditional medicine has not been restricted to treating people; it was also given to horses to improve their immunity.

Whole rosehip powder is made of whole dried rosehips and contains 60 times more vitamin C than citrus fruit. In addition, it is rich in antioxidants and vital minerals, such as iron, calcium, potassium, and magnesium. Rosehip also contains a large amount of folic acid, which is particularly good for breastfeeding women or women trying for a baby. Making your own rosehip powder is simple: dry whole rosehip berries and grind them to a powder.

Makes one shot

1 orange

2 tsp whole rosehip powder

a few frozen strawberries

Rinse the orange and remove the zest, taking care not to remove the nutritious white pith beneath. Blend all the ingredients into a refreshing shot rich in vitamin C!

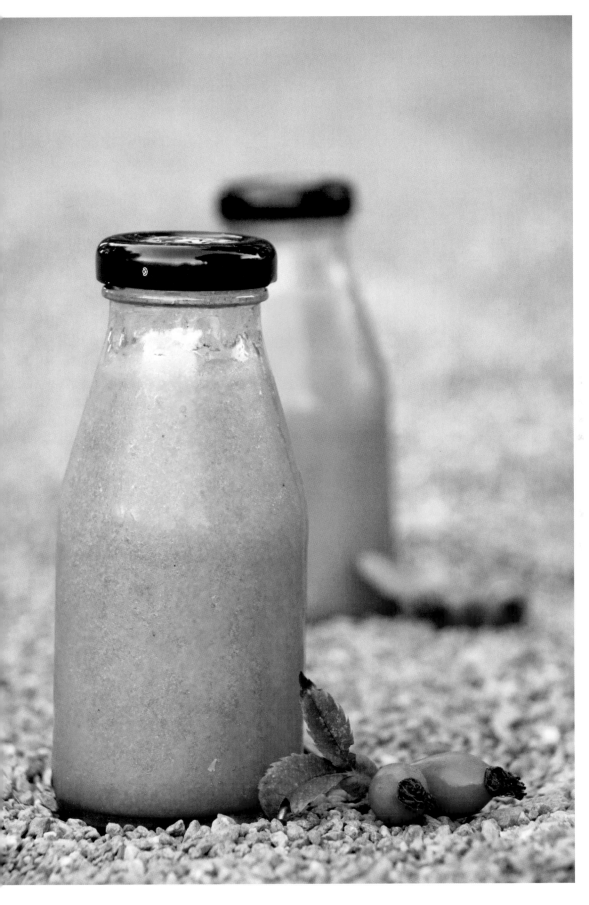

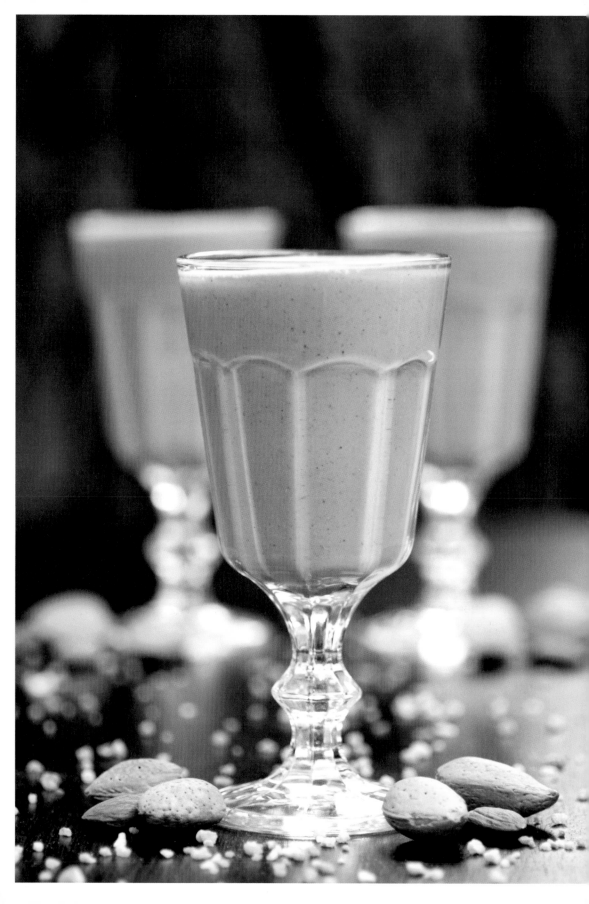

ALMOND CHOCOLATE WITH BANANA AND VANILLA SHAKE

The almond is commonly referred to as a nut, but in the botanical sense, it is a drupe fruit and related, in particular, to plum, peach, and apricot. The actual almond grows as a seed inside the fruit's kernel. The almond is 20 percent protein, contains lots of fiber, and is particularly rich in vitamin E, iron, zinc, calcium, magnesium, potassium, and phosphorus, making it a great ingredient to add to a smoothie after a hard workout at the gym.

You can buy unsweetened almond milk in the store, or you can also make your own by blending almonds or almond butter with water. If you make your own, your milk will contain more almonds than the store-bought version. You will find the recipe for homemade almond milk on page 37. Avoid ready-made, sweetened almond milk as it contains a lot of sugar.

Makes one glass

generous ¾ cup / 200 ml almond milk (or 3 tsp almond butter + 1½ cups / 350 ml water)

1 banana, frozen

2–3 dates, pitted

1 tbsp cocoa powder

1 tsp flaxseed oil (optional)

½ tsp vanilla extract

crushed almonds for garnish

Blend all the ingredients to a smooth consistency. Pour into a glass and sprinkle crushed almonds on top.

CHOCOLATE, DATE, AND TURMERIC SMOOTHIE

Turmeric has anti-inflammatory properties and a strong antioxidant effect against inflammation and damage caused by free radicals (residues formed in the body during oxidation).

Laboratory tests have shown that turmeric prevents atherosclerosis, Alzheimer's disease, and diseases of the pancreas, liver, and the lungs. Turmeric is also said to halt tumor growth in, for example, breast, lung, skin, and prostate cancer.

You should not take large amounts of turmeric if you are pregnant or trying to get pregnant. Always consult your physician if you have any health problems.

Makes one glass

1 banana, frozen

3 dates, pitted

3½ tbsp / 50 ml coconut milk (additive-free)

1 tbsp cold-pressed coconut oil

1 tbsp cacao powder

2 tsp ground turmeric

²⁄₃ cup / 150 ml water

2 oz / 50 g ice (optional)

coconut flakes to garnish

Blend all the ingredients, apart from the ice, to a smooth consistency. Blend in the ice for a frosty smoothie. Serve in a glass and sprinkle coconut flakes on top.

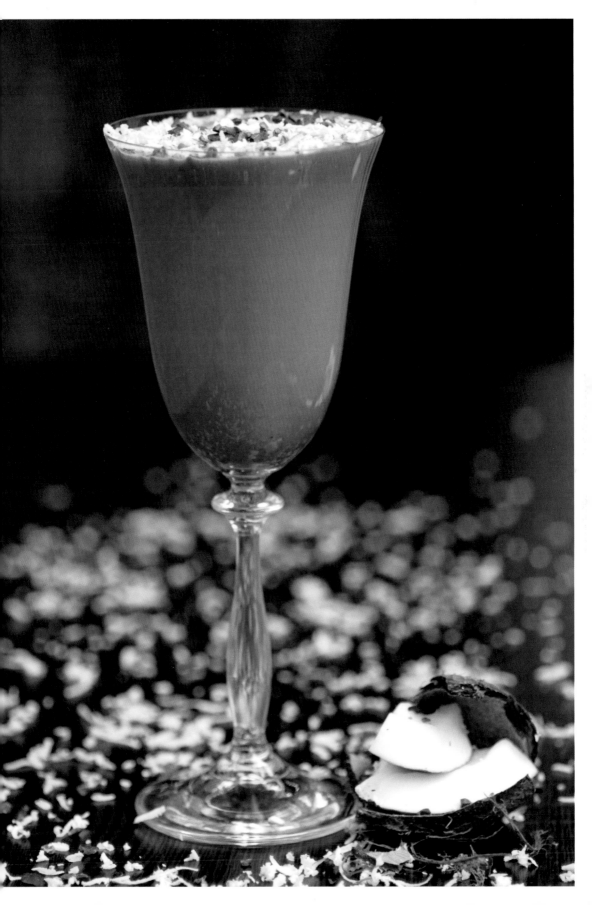

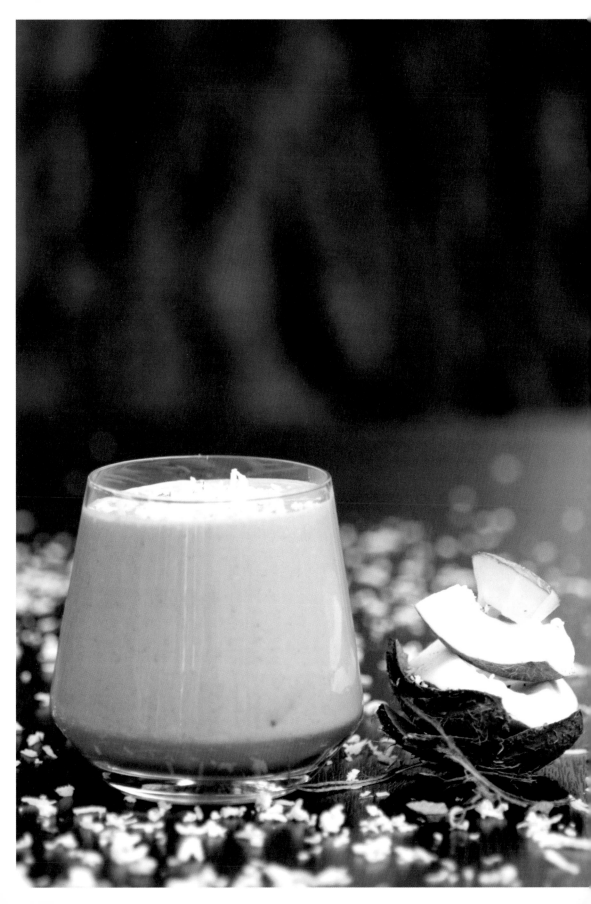

PIÑA CHOCOLADA SHAKE

Coconut oil is one of the healthiest oils in the world. It solidifies at room temperature and turns into liquid at around 75 °F / 24 °C. Some 50 percent of the fat in coconut oil consists of lauric acid, which the body converts to monolauric acid. The latter has antiviral, antifungal, and antibacterial properties. Coconut oil contains the largest amount of lauric acid of all the food products in the world. In addition, it is rich in caprylic acid, which promotes the growth of good intestinal bacteria, is antifungal, and kills parasites in the intestinal tract.

Always buy organic, raw, cold-pressed, unbleached, unrefined, and undeodorized coconut oil. The ingredients section should state 100 percent coconut.

You can use coconut oil for cooking and to make smoothies and desserts, but it is also a handy product for body care. I use coconut oil instead of skin cream.

Makes one glass

7 oz / 200 g pineapple (fresh or frozen)

7 tbsp / 100 ml water

3½ tbsp / 50 ml coconut milk (additive-free)

1 tbsp cold-pressed coconut oil

1 tbsp cocoa powder

1 tbsp cacao nibs

2 oz / 50 g ice (if using fresh pineapple)

coconut flakes to garnish

If using fresh pineapple, remove the leafy crown, cut away the skin, and chop the flesh into small pieces. Blend all the ingredients, apart from the ice, to a smooth consistency. Blend in the ice for a frosty smoothie. Serve in a glass and sprinkle coconut flakes on top.

Good to know: A coconut palm blossoms 13 times a year, yielding an average of 60 coconuts a year. The coconut palm provides us with coconut oil, coconut water, coconut milk, coconut palm sugar, coconut flour, coconut nectar, coconut vinegar, coconut chips, coconut flakes, as well as other things.

PEANUT CHOCOLATE SHAKE

Peanut butter has become popular with athletes and the health conscious thanks to its high content of fiber, protein, healthy fats, minerals, vitamins, and antioxidants. It is also filling. A good peanut butter must be organically produced and consist of at least 99 percent peanuts. It should not contain anything else other than, possibly, a little sea salt. However, unsalted peanut butter is best for smoothies. Stores sell many different brands and there are many that contain both palm oil and sugar—give them a wide berth!

Makes one glass

2 tbsp peanut butter, organic

3 dates, pitted

1 banana, frozen

1 tbsp cocoa powder

generous ¾ cup / 200 ml water

unsalted peanuts, crushed, to garnish

Blend all the ingredients to a smooth consistency. Serve in a glass and sprinkle the crushed peanuts on top.

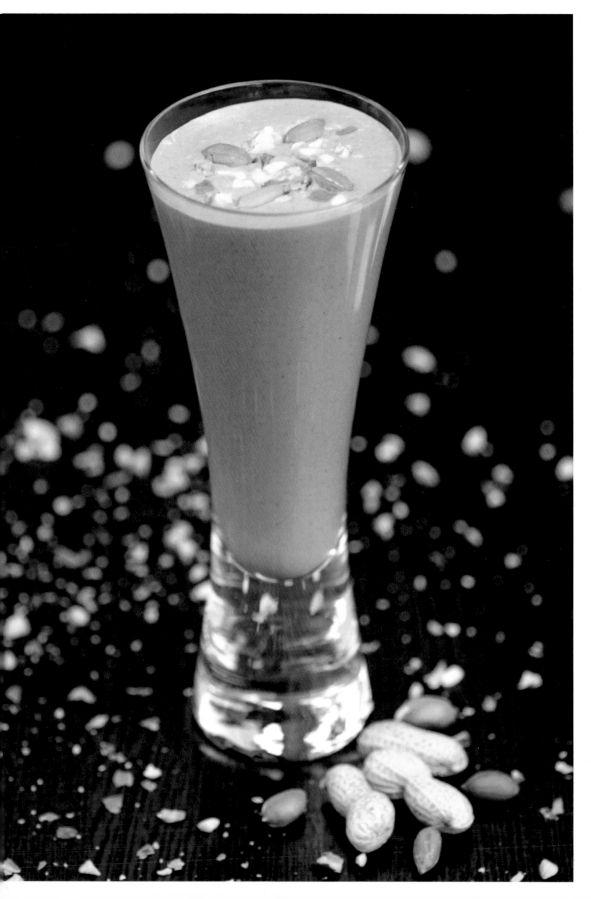

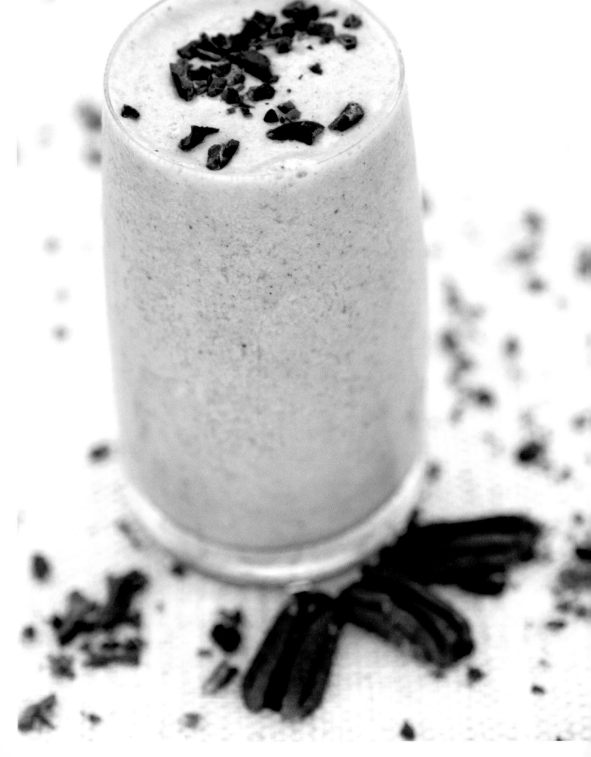

PECAN, DATE, AND COCONUT WATER SHAKE

Coconut water has become quite popular because it is both restorative after a hard workout and a great addition to a smoothie. Coconut water is the clear liquid found in a young, green coconut. Coconut water is 95 percent water, the remainder consisting of nutrients and minerals, such as vitamin B, vitamin C, phosphorus, calcium, and zinc. Coconut water is particularly rich in potassium and is sometimes called "nature's own sports drink."

Coconut water should not be confused with coconut milk, which is produced from the white flesh of a ripe brown coconut. Coconut water freezes very nicely in ice-cube trays. It will keep for half a year in the freezer.

Makes one glass

1 oz / 30 g pecans, soaked for a few hours

3–4 dates, pitted

1 banana

1 tbsp chia seeds

1 tbsp cacao nibs

1¼ cups / 300 ml coconut water, in frozen cubes

Blend all the ingredients to a smooth consistency.

RASPBERRY, COCONUT, AND HEMP SEED SMOOTHIE

Hemp seeds contain high levels of beneficial unsaturated fatty acids, such as omega-3 and omega-6. The seeds are as much as 25 percent protein and are rich in essential amino acids. They also contain high levels of calcium, magnesium, phosphorus, sulfur, carotene, iron, and zinc as well as vitamins E, C, B1, B2, B3, and B6.

Hemp seeds are available in several different forms: shelled, unshelled, or as hemp protein powder, which is excellent as a natural protein supplement.

Makes one glass

1¼ cups / 150 g raspberries, frozen

generous ¾ cup / 200 ml co-conut water, in frozen cubes

7 tbsp / 100 ml coconut milk

1 tbsp coconut flakes, unsweetened

2 tbsp shelled hemp seeds or 1 tbsp hemp protein powder

1 tbsp sunflower seeds

Blend all the ingredients to a smooth consistency.

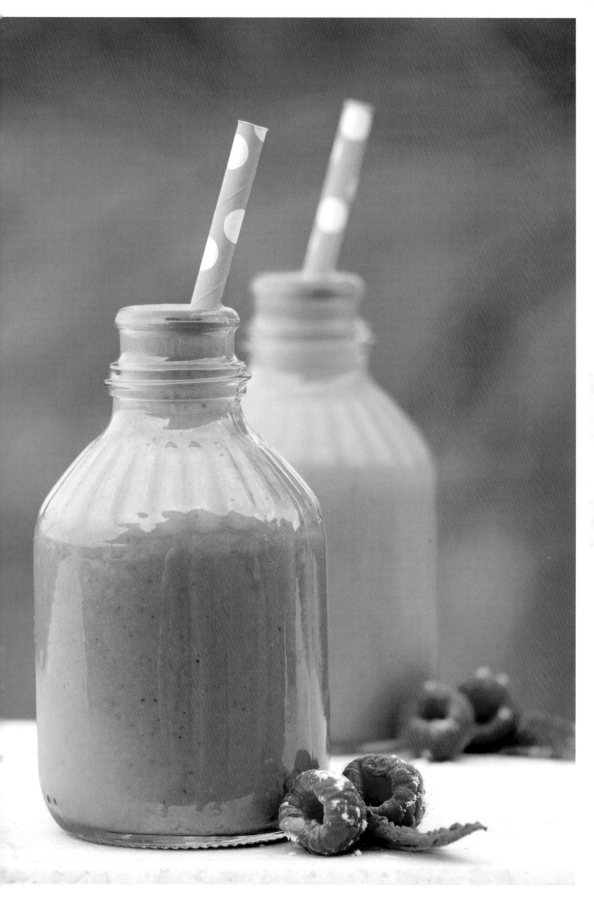

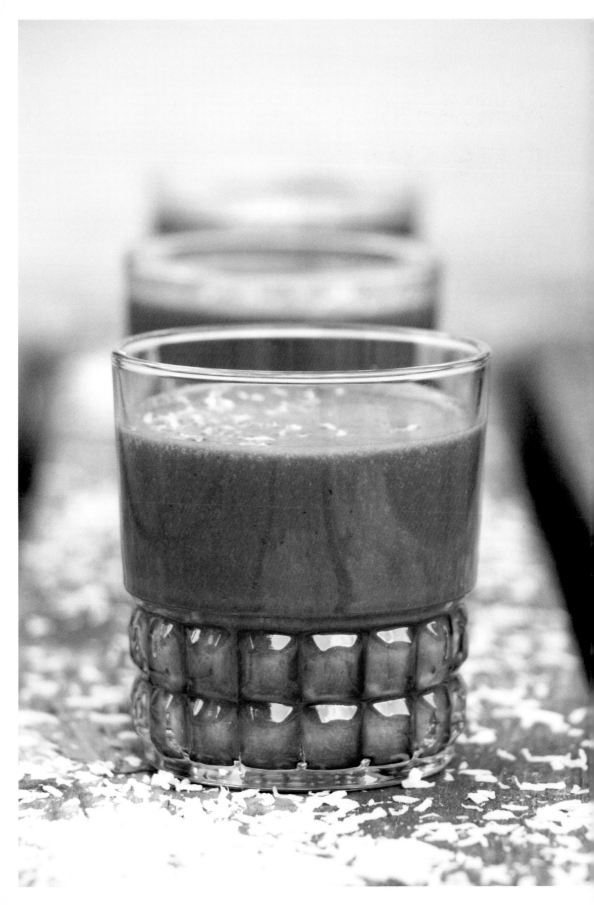

MACA-MOCHA AND DATE SHAKE

The root of the maca plant has traditionally been used for various conditions, e.g. stress-related and hormonal problems, fatigue, malnutrition, and memory difficulties, and for improving immunity. However, maca is best known for being an aphrodisiac and for its fertility-enhancing properties. The maca root contains significant amounts of amino acids, carbohydrates, and minerals, such as calcium, zinc, magnesium, and iron. The maca root also contains vitamins B1, B2, B12, C, and E.

Because of maca's peculiar flavor and its tendency to overpower other flavors easily (it's a little reminiscent of horseradish), it is best to start with a little and increase the quantity to taste. Do combine it with other bold flavors, though!

Makes one glass

1 oz / 30 g cashew nuts, soaked for a few hours

3 dates, pitted

½–1 tbsp maca powder

1 tbsp cacao nibs

1–2 tsp cacao powder

1 tsp coconut flakes

generous ¾ cup / 200 ml water

2 oz / 50 g ice (optional)

Blend all the ingredients, apart from the ice, to a creamy consistency. Blend in the ice for a frosty smoothie. Serve in a large glass with a straw.

AVOCADO, ALMOND, AND ORANGE SHAKE

Avocados are chock full of healthy fats and are said both to prevent wrinkles and to improve brain capacity. Avocado has also been regarded as an aphrodisiac through the ages. In addition to its possible potency-enhancing effect and beneficial monounsaturated fats, avocado contains many nutrients that are good for the blood, liver, heart, skin, and hair. Avocado contains a lot of vitamin E, which makes the skin soft, smooth, and healthy and which gives hair added shine. It's also high in potassium, which helps to regulate blood pressure and is good for muscles. Avocado also contains plenty of fiber, folic acid, and vitamins A, B, and C as well as magnesium.

Makes one glass

1 orange

1 ripe avocado

1 tbsp almond butter

generous ¾ cup / 200 ml almond milk

Rinse the orange and squeeze out the juice. Remove the pit from the avocado and scoop out the flesh. Blend all the ingredients and enjoy a mild-tasting and filling shake.

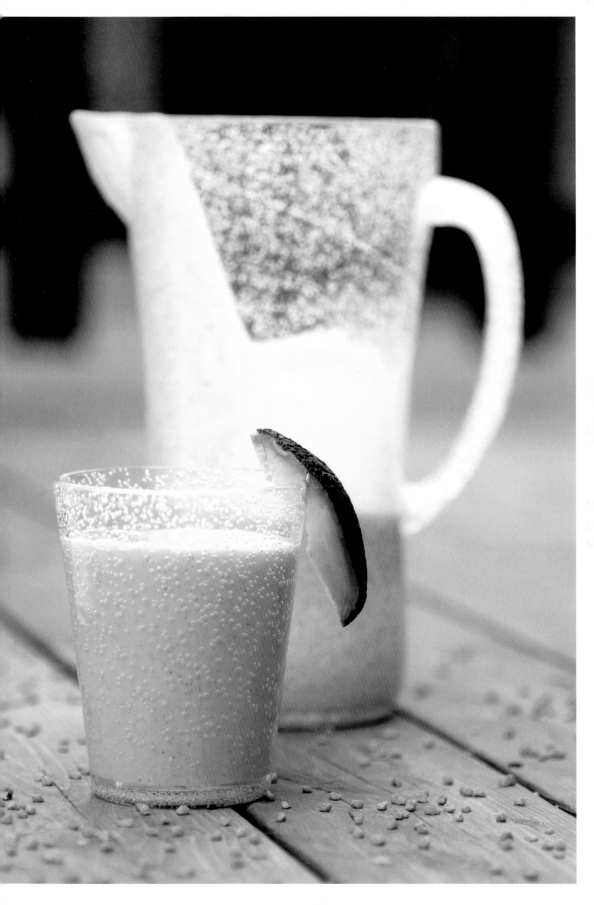

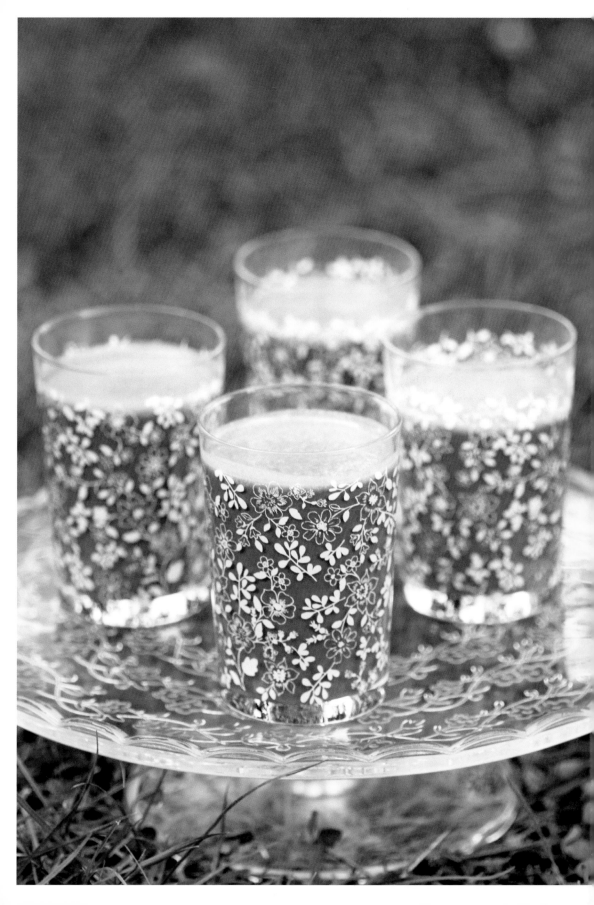

SEED AND NUT CHAI SMOOTHIE

Chai is an Indian spice mix usually drunk as tea. The mixture comprises many different spices, usually containing cardamom, cinnamon, and ginger. Chai is almost always served with milk. Sometimes it is cooked in milk for a more intense flavor.

Makes one glass

1 oz / 30 g cashew nuts, soaked for a few hours (or 2 tbsp cashew butter)

1 tbsp hemp seeds

3 dates, pitted

1 tsp cacao nibs

1 tsp chia seeds

1 tsp ground cinnamon

1 tsp ground ginger

½ tsp ground cardamom

1 tsp raw cacao powder

generous ¾ cup / 200 ml coconut water

1 banana, frozen

2 oz / 50 g ice (optional)

Blend all the ingredients, apart from the frozen banana and ice, to a smooth consistency. Add the banana and ice and blend for a frosty smoothie.

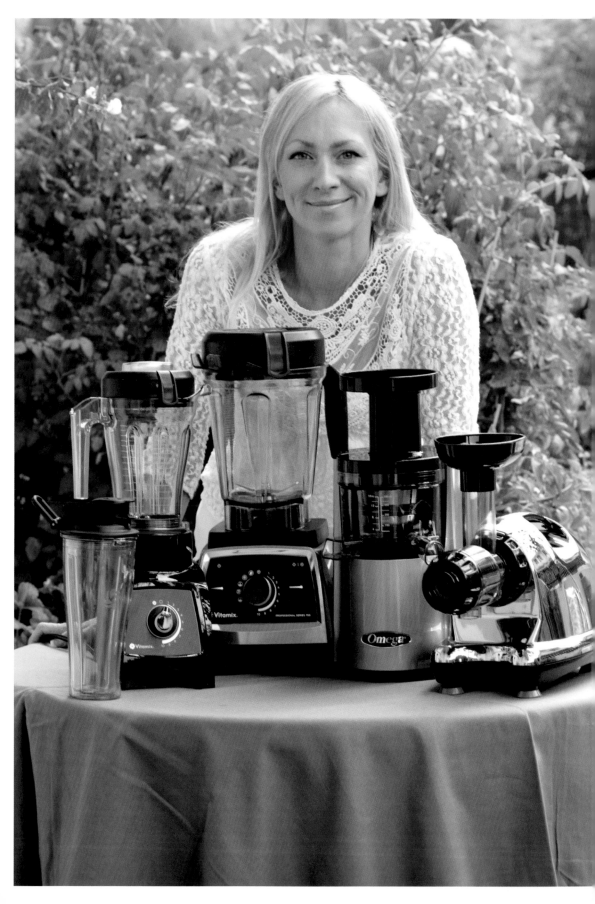

RECIPE INDEX

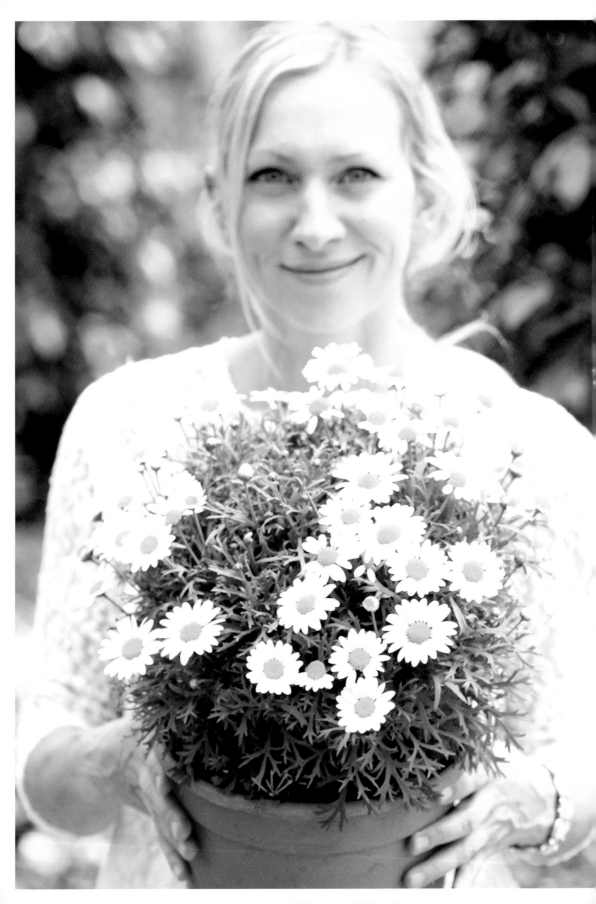

ACKNOWLEDGEMENTS

I would like to thank...

... my beloved daughter Jasmine for brightening every day of my life.

... my beloved husband and agent, Stefan Lindström, who has always believed in me and my crazy ideas.

... my dear brother, Alan Maranik, for the book's incredibly appealing design. It's always fun to work with you.

... my editor, Eva Stjerne, for her fantastic linguistic input.

... Vitamix and Carl Uggla at Lindenbaum Agenturer for all the Vitamix blenders. It's amazing what these powerhouses can do!

... Herbert Ullmann, Florian Ullmann, Lars Pietzschmann, Isabel Weiler, and everyone at h.f.ullmann Publishing and Tandem Verlag for working to publish my books throughout the world.

Abbreviations and Quantities

1 oz = 1 ounce = 28 grams
1 lb = 1 pound = 16 ounces 1
1 cup = approx. 5–8 ounces* (see below)
1 cup = 8 fl uid ounces = 250 milliliters (liquids)
2 cups = 1 pint (liquids) = 15 milliliters (liquids)
8 pints = 4 quarts = 1 gallon (liquids)
1 g = 1 gram = 1/1000 kilogram = 5 ml (liquids)
1 kg = 1 kilogram = 1000 grams = 2¼ lb
l l = 1 liter = 1000 milliliters (ml) = 1 quart
125 milliliters (ml) = approx. 8 tablespoons = ½ cup
1 tbsp = 1 level tablespoon = 15–20 g* (depending on density) = 15 milliliters (liquids)
1 tsp = 1 level teaspoon = 3–5 g * (depending on density) = 5 ml (liquids)

*The weight of dry ingredients varies significantly depending on the density factor, e.g. 1 cup of flour weighs less than 1 cup of butter. Quantities in ingredients have been rounded up or down for convenience, where appropriate. Metric conversions may therefore not correspond exactly. It is important to use either American or metric measurements within a recipe.

The purpose of the recipes and advice in this book is simply to give guidance on quality nutrition and how to increase your energy. If you have a medical condition you should consult your doctor.

© Eliq Maranik and Stevali Production
Original title: *Detox & viktminskning med SMOOTHIES & JUICER*
ISBN 978-91-86287-73-3

Text: Eliq Maranik
Photos: Eliq Maranik and Stefan Lindström, except pp. 8, 14, 18, 23, 30, 36, 41: iStockphoto
Layout: Eliq Maranik and Alan Maranik/Stevali Production
Editor: Eva Stjerne Ord & Form

© for the English edition: h.f.ullmann publishing GmbH

Translation from Swedish: Casper Sare in association with First Edition Translations Ltd, Cambridge, UK
Coverphotos: Eliq Maranik and Stefan Lindström

Overall responsibility for production: h.f.ullmann publishing GmbH, Potsdam, Germany

Printed in Poland, 2015

ISBN 978-3-8480-0882-7

10 9 8 7 6 5 4 3 2 1
X IX VIII VII VI V IV III II I

www.ullmann-publishing.com
newsletter@ullmann-publishing.com
facebook.com/ullmann.social

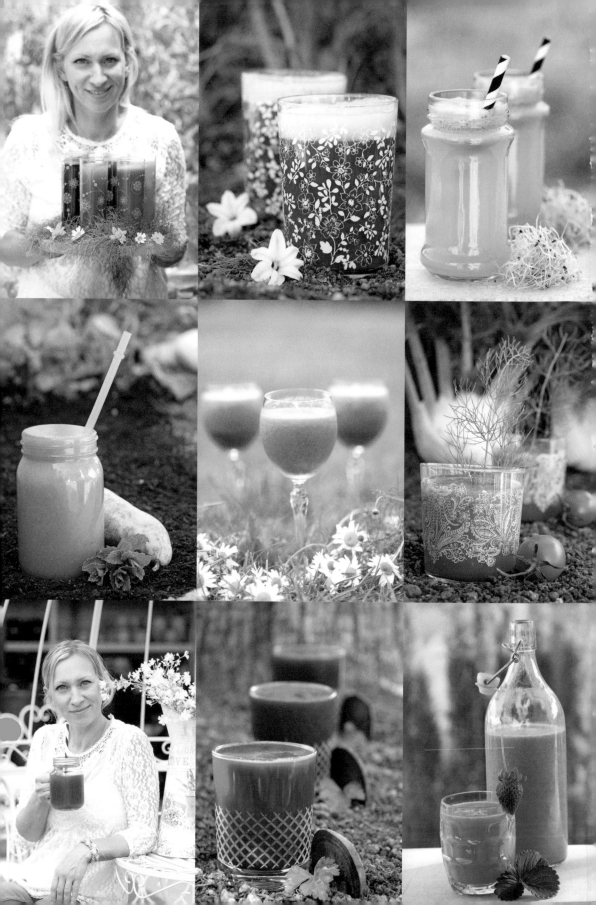